"*MOOOOve Over Milk* is the most thorough, yet concise, argument for cow's milk being the most serious health hazard facing the people of our nation."

- **John McDougall, MD**
  Health speaker, TV and radio personality, and author of The McDougall Plan, McDougall's Medicine, *and numerous articles.*

"I'm not a nutrition researcher, but I'm a parent advisor, and I want to pass the word to parents that cow's milk from the carton has definite faults for some babies. *MOOOOve Over Milk* shows those faults clearly, concisely, and in a very readable manner."

- **Benjamin Spock, MD**
  Pediatrician and author of Baby and Child Care

"I give *MOOOOve Over Milk* an A! It's a big eye-opener and very well put together."

- **Hans Diehl, DrHSc, MPH**
  Former Pritikin researcher, speaker, TV and radio personality, president of Lifestyle Medicine Institute, and author of To Your Health *and* Dynamic Living

"Cow's milk. I don't drink it anymore. *MOOOOve Over Milk* reinforces my determination to be dairy free. It is scientifically sound, reveals the latest research, and exposes a kitchenful of dairy deceptions. The charts, graphs, and illustrations make the information easy to understand and remember. *MOOOOve Over Milk* will move into my library beside my other health classics. I would highly recommend this book to anyone striving for optimum health."

- **DeWitt S. Williams, EdD, MPH, CHES**
  Director, GC/NAD Health Department

"I couldn't put this book down! Cow's milk is an unnatural source of foreign protein and excessive fat. It contributes to most of the chronic diseases which lead to premature disability and death. Also, milk is not a solution to osteoporosis, it is part of the problem."

- **Charles R. Attwood, MD**
  Pediatrician and author of Dr. Attwood's Low-Fat Prescription [illegible] The Gold Stan-

"Milk and other dairy products will support life and perhaps even make you fat, but they also promote and produce chronic diseases, particularly in the middle-aged and the elderly. Advertising of milk products has been misleading and mind-binding. The bias of the seller and those financially supporting the dairy industry must be resisted. That's what *MOOOOve Over Milk* does! The livelihood of one industry is far less important than the health of the nation."

- **Richard W. Hubbard, PhD, CNS**
  Associate Professor of Pathology, Biochemistry and Nutrition, Loma Linda University; author of **Diet to Alter the Disease Process: A Review of the Effects of Protein and Fat on Disease.**

"If you still believe that milk 'does a body good,' read *MOOOOve Over Milk*—and be prepared for a tall, cold drink of reality. Clearly and courageously, the authors present the evidence of the health threats posed by modern dairy products. Advice worth hearing—and a warning worth heeding."

- **Michael A. Klaper, MD**
  Speaker, researcher, and author of **Vegan Nutrition: Pure and Simple**

(See back of cover for more professional endorsements of ***MOOOOve Over Milk***.)

NOTE: Citizens of most Western nations come in contact daily with advertisements praising the virtues of milk and milk products. But, for the most part, they're hearing just one side of the story. While evidence shows that drinking milk may have some benefits, new medical studies show that it can also present health risks—some potentially serious. It is important, then, for consumers to be aware of the potential problems with milk. That is why this book was written—to present "the other side of the story." Research into milk's potential role in increasing the risk for certain diseases is onging. This book presents some of the evidence gathered to date. Carefully consider it. The information presented in ***MOOOOve Over Milk*** has been obtained from respected, reliable scientific and journalistic sources. Although great care has been taken to ensure the accuracy of the information presented, the authors and publisher cannot be responsible for the accuracy of the original sources cited. Read ***MOOOOve Over Milk*** for yourself. It provides you with information that will help you make a more informed, intelligent decision about your milk consumption habits. Before implementing any changes, always consult with your health care provider.

The Authors.

Foreword

by

Charles R. Attwood, MD
T. Colin Campbell, PhD

From vastly different backgrounds, viewpoints, and experiences, we have reached the same conclusion: Milk is not the wholesome food that most Americans have been led to believe it is. Furthermore, considerable scientific evidence suggests that milk is partially responsible for much of the present epidemic of chronic disease and premature deaths in North America and other Western nations. One of us, a practicing pediatrician for 36 years, has seen first hand this morbidity among patients for more than two generations. The other, a scientist in an academic setting, has observed these same disease processes in the laboratory and the famed China Health Project he directs.

But most individuals have been led to believe that milk and dairy products are not only wholesome, but are absolutely necessary for adequate calcium and protein. Who should they believe? The "dairy dilemma" is encountered most frequently by families trying to reduce their saturated fat and animal protein intake. They've read that both may increase the risk of heart disease and many kinds of cancers. But they worry about their calcium balance and bone density if milk, one of the chief sources of saturated fat and animal protein, is discontinued.

Why is this paranoia so common among Americans? The milk-protein-calcium-bone density myth has been created and perpetuated by intense lobbying of the dairy industry throughout the lifetimes of most adults living today. While in kindergarten and grade school, a great number of the nutrition teaching aids were supplied by the National Dairy Council. As a result, parents, teachers, doctors, lawyers, judges, and significantly, members of congress, have grown up with the not unbiased view that milk is both wholesome and necessary to the daily diet. For several generations, the Council's most effective campaign tool has been to link milk with calcium and bone density.

To further confuse the consumer, the dairy industry has fortified milk and infant formulas with vitamin D, which is necessary for proper calcium absorption. But vitamin D is self-manufactured in adequate amounts by exposure to as little as 10-15 minutes of sunlight about three times a week. Even among those who get no sunlight, such as the totally disabled, vitamin D may be obtained from supplements or fortified cereals. So fortified cow's milk isn't necessary.

The dairy industry hasn't been telling us the truth about the connection between milk and strong bones. Calcium balance, the relationship between the intake and loss of calcium, determines bone density, primarily during the growing years and early adulthood. If one has a good bone density by the age of 30, it will usually last a lifetime for those consuming a balanced plant-based diet and remaining physically active.

Milk and other dairy products, although rich in calcium, are excessively high in animal protein, which has been shown to create calcium loss from the bones through the urinary tract. The evidence for this loss is substantial .

A 1994 National Institutes of Health Consensus Statement formulated by an expert panel concluded that calcium balance and bone density depended at least 3O percent on the ratio of calcium intake to loss, not on calcium intake alone.

But this isn't a new idea. A report in *Science* magazine in 1986, stated that evidence was accumulating that calcium intake ***alone*** is not related to bone density and osteoporosis.

This may explain why countries with the highest consumption of dairy products also have the highest incidence of osteoporosis—and why bone fracture rates in these societies are more closely tied to ***excess*** protein consumption than to ***inadequate*** calcium consumption. Exceptions exist, but it's interesting that countries with the highest animal protein consumption are the very countries with a higher than normal recommended daily allowance (RDA) for calcium.

Higher animal protein consumption would require a higher intake of calcium to offset the adverse effects of the extra protein!

The RDA of calcium in the United States is now 1,200 mg. daily. But the World Health Organization, which concentrates on countries where dairy intake is minimal or nonexistent, recommends just 500 mg. for children and 800 mg. for adults. Studies among humans have shown that these much lower levels of calcium intake can sustain good calcium balance and good bone health for all age groups.

To further illustrate the relationship of protein consumption to calcium balance, let's consider two cultures at opposite ends of the protein spectrum. Elderly South African Bantu women, who consume a very low protein diet (5O grams daily, compared with 91 grams for Americans) and only 450 mg. calcium daily, have little or no osteoporosis despite the calcium drain of nursing an average of 10 children.

On the other hand, Eskimos, who are very physically active, consume a very high protein diet (250-400 grams, mostly from fish), and have a calcium intake of over 2,000 mg. daily. Yet they have the highest rate of osteoporosis in the world! So the high protein content of milk—yes, even skim milk—could well undermine its high calcium content.

Now, let's take a new look at milk and dairy products as a calcium source, regardless of their protein content. It isn't as good as we've been told it is. Here's why: The chart below shows that calcium content expressed as mg. per 100 calories, instead of per gram, puts milk and cheese at the bottom of the list and green vegetables at the top! *(See chart on the next page.)*

Calcium in Milligrams per 100 Calories	
Arugula	1,300
Watercress	800
Turnip greens	650
Collard greens	548
Mustard greens	490
Spinach	450
Broccoli	387
Swiss cheese	250
Milk (2%)	245
Green onions	240
Okra	213
Cabbage	196
Whole milk	190
Cheddar cheese	179
American cheese	160

At first glance, one may conclude, "But I would have to eat so much more broccoli or turnip greens to get adequate calcium." Not so! Individuals eating a plant-based diet generally consume as many or more total calories as do meat and dairy-eaters. In other words, adequate amounts of vegetables are better sources of calcium than milk and cheese.

But wait! Don't many green vegetables contain oxalic acid, which reduces the absorption of their calcium? This too, it seems, has been exaggerated by the dairy lobby.

A 1990 report in the American Journal of Clinical Nutrition concluded that greens such as broccoli and kale have a high level of calcium which is absorbed at least as well as the calcium in milk. Contrary to what we've heard, excellent calcium balance on a nondairy diet is easily attained because all vegetables and legumes contain calcium which, collectively, is more than adequate for our needs.

Simply put, it's the whole plate that counts, not just a side glass or serving of concentrated calcium, such as milk or cheese. And the plant calcium is much more likely to stay in the bones where it belongs, unlike much of the calcium from high-protein dairy products.

Now it begins to make sense. In societies where the most protein is consumed, the calcium requirement for good bone density and protection against osteoporosis may be UNATTAINABLY high, without supplements—it's a Catch-22. But for the majority of the world's population, and among those consuming a plant-based diet in Western countries, calcium requirements for normal bone density are easily obtained without milk or other dairy products. Milk, it now seems clear, is not the solution to the malady of poor bone density. Rather, it's almost certainly a part of the problem.

What about strong, durable teeth? Ironically, tooth decay among children has been far more related to the bathing of infant teeth by milk than to the lack of milk in the diet. The absolute worst decay pediatricians and dentists see is known as the "milk bottle syndrome," where infants fall asleep with a bottle of milk in their mouths.

Human epidemiological studies have strongly related animal protein consumption to various cancers. Of all animal protein, there is strong experimental evidence that casein, the principal protein of milk, is especially capable of promoting cancer development. Controlled studies have shown that in cancer-prone laboratory mice, the amount of casein in their diet is directly related to the appearance of experimental tumors. When the dietary casein is withdrawn or replaced by plant proteins, further cancer development is either arrested or reversed!

What are the other problems with milk and dairy products? The majority of practicing pediatric allergists insist that more than half of their patients are allergic to one or more of milk's more than 2 dozen proteins. Their allergy symptoms include eczema, asthma, middle ear infections, sinus infections, rhinitis, gastroenteritis, and allergic colitis—conditions responsible for 80-90 percent of doctor's office visits.

And that number may be a conservative estimate, since circulating plasma immunoglobulin G and immunoglobulin M antibodies to various milk proteins can be detected in nearly all individuals who consume dairy products. But is this allergy reaction something new? Not at all.

Hippocrates (460-370 B.C.) called attention to adverse effects of cow's milk in his day! He wrote that it could cause skin rashes and gastric problems. His may be among the first references in history to lactose intolerance, a very common problem in our world today.

If heart disease, stroke, cancer, and everyday allergies aren't enough to think about, how about industrial pollutants? There is good evidence that the highly toxic compound dioxin, a byproduct of burning waste and paper mill production, finds its way into most large animals. One of the only ways dioxin can be eliminated from the body, other than by extensive fasting, is through lactation. So, if a milk cow has dioxin in its body, it will certainly be in the cow's milk, too. Think about it.

Still another worry with milk protein is its uncanny ability to elevate blood cholesterol. In both human and animal studies, some published almost 100 years ago, both casein and lactalbumin (another milk protein) have been shown to substantially increase blood cholesterol levels.

Even some human studies show that the effect of milk protein-intake on blood cholesterol is more substantial than the effect of either saturated fat or dietary cholesterol intake! This factor could explain why cholesterol levels are not easily controlled by simply having patients switch from red meat to fish or poultry, or from whole milk to skim milk.

Moooove Over Milk gives the reader important information about all of these concerns and many more. The book addresses other important risks incurred by persons consuming dairy products. These include lactose intolerance, intestinal bleeding and anemia, contamination by bacteria and other infectious agents, antibiotics, hormones, pesticides, and the relationship of cow's milk consumption during infancy to the later development of insulin-dependent diabetes.

Mooove Over Milk is a resource of information long feared and dreaded by the dairy industry.

And now it's here!

Some of the information in this foreword came from the following references:

1. NIH Conference Statement, 1994 June 6-8;12(4);1-31.
2. Science 1986;233:519-520.
3. Clinical Science 1974;27:916-925.
4. American Journal of Clinical Nutrition 1965;16:327.
5. American Journal of Clinical Nutrition 1974;27:916-925.
6. Pediatric Annals 1997;26:244-250.
7. Journal of Pediatrics 1992;121:S64-S71.

Charles R. Attwood, M.D., F.A.A.P., a pediatrician in Crowley, Louisiana, is the author of *Dr. Attwood's Low-Fat Prescription For Kids, One Diet for the Whole Family* (Viking) and the new audio series, *The Gold Standard Diet, How to Live to be 100* (Knowledge Products). His articles (winners of two national awards) and interviews have appeared in hundreds of national and international publications.

T. Colin Campbell, Ph.D., is the Jacob Gould Schurman Professor of Nutritional Biochemistry at Cornell University. He is the director of the China, Oxford, Cornell Project on Diet, Lifestyle, and Disease Characteristics. His data, according to the *New York Times*, will continue to produce valuable information for the next 50 years.

Table of Contents

Because this book is not divided into chapters, we have provided you with this guide to help you find information quickly. The charts box below lists pages where full-page or quarter-page charts or information blocks are found. The various large quotation blocks found on each page are not listed here, as there are too many to list.

Introduction 1
Human vs. cow milk 6
Milk and infants 8
Milk and diabetes 12
Milk and allergy 20
Lactose intolerance 22
Milk and cataracts 24
Milk and heart disease 26
Milk and bone health 33
Milk and protein 41
Protein and pH 45
Incomplete protein? 50
Milk and cancer 54
Milk and lactose 58
Vitamin D 60
Milk and leukemia 64
Milk and BLV 68, 75
Milk and MS 71
Milk and AIDS 77
Say cheese? 79
Milk and "bugs" 84
Milk and listeria 86
Milk and Crohn's 90
Milk and drugs 95
Milk and rBGH 99
Milk and mad cow disease 103
Animal rendering 109
Milking soy cows? 115

Charts

Protein comparison *7*
Milk's added extras *9*
Cow-lorie counting *18*
Diabetes *13,19*
Are you intolerant? *23*
Girth control *31*
Calcium needs *33*
Osteoporosis update *39*
Protein needs *43*
The incomplete story *47*
Food calcium levels *51*
Cancer update *57*
Allergy update *72*
Beware of the cow *73*
Cream of the crop? *85*
More on mycobacterium *97*
rBGH update *101*
Mad cow update *109*
B-ware *113*
Udder update *119*
Dairy-free recipes *125*
Ultimate update *132*

Introduction

You've probably heard the slogan: "*Milk has something for everybody.*" Besides calcium and other minerals and vitamins, what else *could* milk have for you?

There is one thing dairy products have more of than any other food I can think of:

contamination.

John A. McDougall, MD

Popular speaker, TV personality, and author of *The McDougall Plan* and *McDougall's Medicine*

Introduction

When people talk with their physician about removing milk and dairy products from their diet, many times the very first question they ask is:

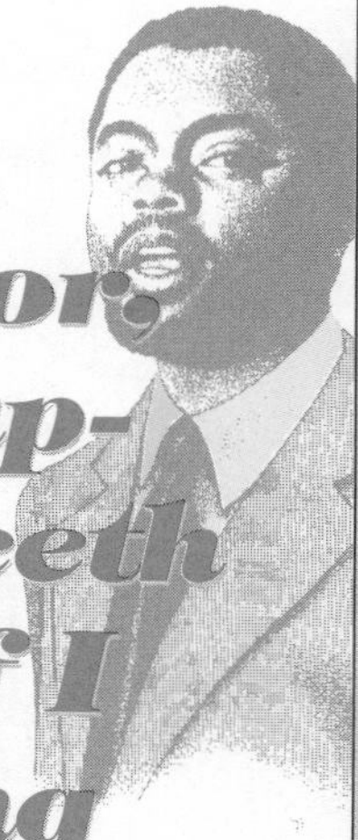

"But doctor, what will happen to my teeth and bones if I stop drinking milk?" Nothing. Nothing that wouldn't have happened anyway."

Frank A. Oski, MD

Former Chairman, Department of Pediatrics, State University of New York, Syracuse

That fact may surprise many because we've all been told that milk is a good food for preventing osteoporosis. But scientific studies prove that:

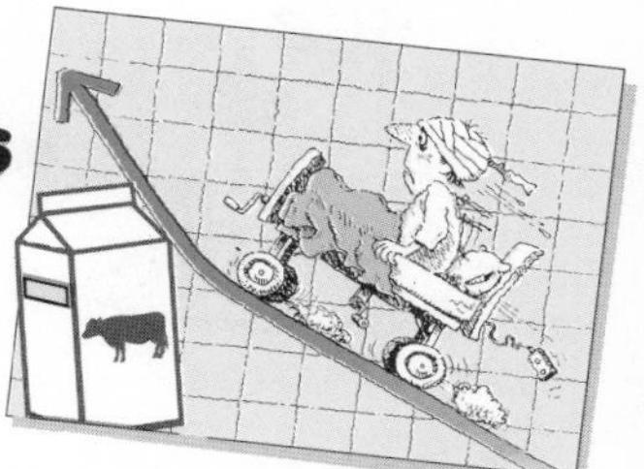

"Cultures with the highest milk consumption have the highest osteoporosis rates, a disease rarely found in non-milk-drinking cultures."

Hans Diehl, Dr HSc
***Dynamic Living*, p. 108**

Surprised? Read on! The information in this book just may moooooooove you away from dairy products—

FOR GOOD!

> **"Perhaps when the public is educated as to the hazards of milk, only calves will be left to drink the real thing."**
>
> *Don't Drink Your Milk, p. 100*

It's hard to imagine a home in the United States without a car in the in the garage, a VCR by every TV, an answering machine in the den, a microwave in the kitchen, and a gallon of milk in the fridge. Maybe two gallons.

Milk. The very word conjures feelings of warmth, security, health, and vitality. Not only mother's milk, but cow's milk, too, is associated with love, American innocence, apple pie, strong bones, and athletic prowess.

It is true that there is no match for mother's milk. Breast-fed babies of healthy mothers generally have a nutritional and immunological edge over formula-fed babies, and may have a lower risk for certain cancers later in life.[1]

But the use of cow's milk for human consumption has come under close scrutiny in the last 15 to 20 years. Its value for regular human consumption is being questioned in an increasing number of medical studies.

Evidence continues to surface linking cow's milk consumption to mineral deficiencies in babies, illnesses caused by lactose intolerance, allergies, juvenile diabetes, various cancers, heart disease, cataracts, and numerous bacterial and viral diseases. Even the claim that milk is a great food to build strong bones is being fractured by strong contrary scientific evidence.

Touching A Sacred Cow?

Because of concerns about milk contamination from hormones, pesticides, and antibiotics, many consumers are considering putting milk out to pasture, and turning to milk alternatives, such as soy, oat, nut, or rice milks as a safe, healthy replacement for dairy milk.

Any investigation of dairy products will certainly touch on some sacred cows. While space will not permit us to present all the evidence, we will skim the cream of the newest information available.

Of all mammals, human milk has the lowest protein content and the lowest ratio of casein to whey.

Proceedings of the Society for Experimental Biology and Medicine 1990:193;143

What are some differences between bovine (cow) and human milk? Milks are complex mixtures containing protein, fat, lactose (sugar), vitamins, minerals, and other biologic agents such as enzymes, cells, hormones, and immunoglobulins (protein-like antibodies).

But cow's milk is different from human milk in some very significant ways. While it is similar to human milk in its fat content, cow's milk contains almost four times more protein than human milk (3.5 grams/deciliter [g/dl] for a cow vs. just 0.9 g/dl for humans).[2]

Both cow and human milk contain two types of protein, casein and whey. But cow's milk is 82% casein and 18% whey,[3] while human milk is mostly whey protein. The casein content in human milk is about 20%,[4] but can go as high as 45% while a mother is nursing.[4]

Human casein also differs structurally from bovine casein in that it contains less calcium and phosphorus. Because of that difference, human casein forms softer, more digestible curds in the stomach.[1] But why would that matter?

Cattle produce a digestive enzyme called rennin, which curdles the large protein molecules and helps them enter the nursing calf's system slowly. Because humans lack such a

Comparing protein content of Cow & other milks

Notice that the more protein in a mother's milk, the faster a baby doubles its birth weight.

Species	% calories from protein	Time taken to double birth weight
Human	*5*	**180 days**
Mare	*11*	**60 days**
Cow	*15*	**47 days**
Goat	*17*	**19 days**
Dog	*30*	**8 days**
Cat	*40*	**7 days**
Rat	*49*	**4 days**

A Diet for a New America, p. 175

digestive aid, large amounts of casein are delivered to the small intestine and may be absorbed into the body without being properly digested.[1] This incomplete digestion can lead to some serious troubles, which will be discussed in a bit more detail later in this book.

Have You "Herd" This?

These and other problems led the authors of one study to conclude: "The consequences of bovine milk consumption are diverse, some of which are potentially deleterious...What is good for the goose may be good for the gander, but what is good for the cow could be harmful to the human."[1]

Other researchers agree. Feeding cow's milk to infants poses several "nutritional hazards,"[5] including gastrointestinal blood loss, and copper and zinc deficiency.[5] Even though zinc concentrations are higher in cow's milk than human milk, the zinc in human milk may be easier for humans to assimilate than the zinc in cow's milk or infant formulas.[5]

Why are zinc and copper important? Zinc is essential for prostate gland function, the growth of reproductive organs, for protein synthesis, collagen (connective tissue) formation, and proper immune function.

Among its many other jobs, copper aids in the formation of bones, hemoglobin (the oxygen-carrying component of your red blood cells), and red blood cells. It also works in cooperation with zinc and vitamin C to form elastin, another type of connective tissue. Obviously, proper zinc and copper absorption are vi-

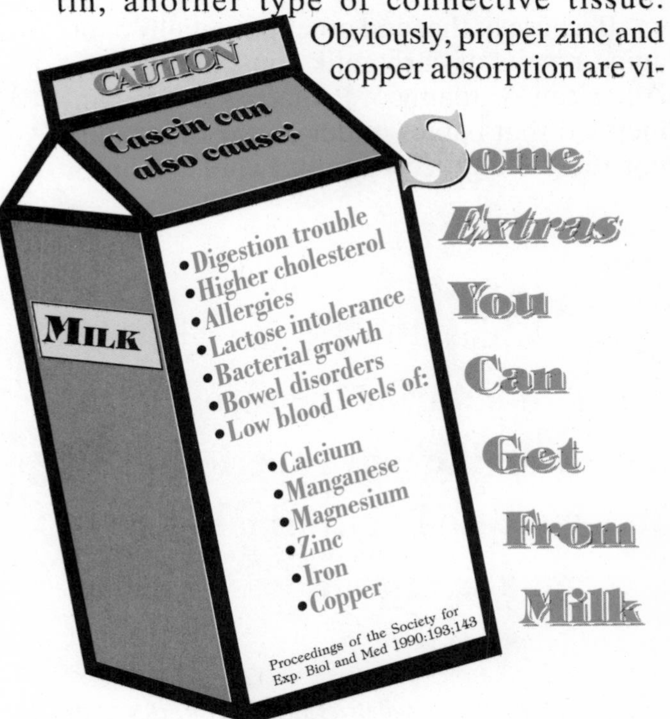

tally important for maintaining good health. But there's more to consider.

According to the American Academy of Pediatrics, cow's milk is not the best food for infants because it contains too much sodium, potassium, and protein, too little iron and linoleic acid, and not enough of vitamins C and E.[6]

Because of that and other potentially damaging results of early milk consumption, the American Academy of Pediatrics has recommended that babies under 1 year old should not receive any cow's milk (whole, skim or

Babies who are fed whole cow's milk during the second six months of life may experience a 30% increase in intestinal blood loss and a significant loss of iron in their stools.

Pediatrics 1992;89(6):1105-1109

"We should strive to use foods... that meet the nutrient needs of the older infant..., yet avoid toxicity. Cow milk simply does not meet this standard of quality."

Journal of Pediatric Gastroenterology and Nutrition 1993;16(1):2

reduced-fat) or any products that contain whole cow's milk.[6]

Among other things, the Academy stated: "The studies of the past 7 years demonstrate the difficulty of providing a balanced diet for older infants when whole cow's milk (WCM) replaces breast milk or iron-fortified formula.

"Nutrients from commonly consumed solid foods do not complement nutrients from WCM; rather, they exaggerate the deficiencies (iron, linoleic acid, and vitamin E) and excesses (sodium, potassium, chloride, and protein) in the infant's diet....

"Recent studies suggest that iron deficiency

in early childhood may lead to long-term changes in behavior that may not be reversed even with iron supplementation."[6]

On the Let's Eat! video ***MOOOOve Over Milk***, Charles Attwood, MD, a pediatrician, lecturer, author, and consultant to Dr. Benjamin Spock, tells how milk has affected his pediatric patients, and what happened when they stopped drinking it. It's fascinating. More about the milk video later.

MOOOOving To Diabetes?

Recently, several studies have implicated the early use of cow's milk as a significant risk factor for developing type I insulin dependent

(Continued on page 14)

Drinking cow's milk may weaken immune function in children and lead to problems with recurring infections.

Nature 1978;272(5654):632

About 1 million Americans have type I, or juvenile diabetes. Some researchers say the strongest environmental factors are:

- ★ **Early dietary exposure to cow's milk**
- ★ **Short duration of breast feeding**
- ★ **High milk intake after age 9, or at diabetes onset**
- ★ **Recent infection**
- ★ **Attending day care before age 3**

These new studies, and more than 20 well-documented previous ones, have prompted one researcher to say the link between milk and juvenile diabetes is "very solid."

Diabetes Care 1994;17(12);1381-1388
Medical Tribune 1995;36(3)

A young age at introduction of dairy products and high milk consumption during childhood may increase the child's risk of developing juvenile diabetes.

Diabetologia 1994;37(4):381-387

diabetes mellitus (IDDM), or juvenile diabetes.[7-12]

Many respected researchers believe that the protein in cow's milk is able to trigger the human body to permanently destroy its own insulin-producing beta cells in the pancreas.[8,9,10]

A recent Canadian study reported a strong relationship between early exposure to cow's milk and the development of insulin-dependent diabetes.[8]

In another study, 142 children with IDDM all had highly elevated serum concentrations of antibodies against the bovine whey protein.[9] That means their bodies had "seen" the whey protein as an invading disease "bug" and had begun to manufacture antibodies to fight against it.

How can such a drastic reaction happen in the body? There is a 17-amino acid peptide chain commonly found in the insulin-producing beta cells of the pancreas that is almost identical to a 17-amino acid peptide chain found in cow's milk.[9]

The Nearsighted Pit Bulls

In some children, the body "sees" that amino acid peptide chain in milk as an invading pathogen, or antigenic protein, which then produces antibodies against it. These same

Alive and Kicking!

Reports that early consumption of cow's milk could cause juvenile diabetes created quite a stir in the medical community. Studies soon appeared that apparently refuted those early findings. Several recent studies that reconfirm the milk-diabetes link, however, caused one researcher to write:

"The cow's milk story remains alive and kicking."

Lancet 1996;348(9032):905-906

antibodies then attack, like "nearsighted pit bulls,"[10] not only the whey protein, but the insulin-producing beta cells in the child's pancreas, destroying their ability to produce life-sustaining insulin forever.[9]

According to Michael Dosch, MD, professor of pediatrics and immunology at the Hospital for Sick Children in Toronto, "In principle, it would be simple to prevent the exposure to cow's milk in the first three months of life. If we are right, it could be the beginning of the end of type I diabetes."[10]

Other researchers agree. One group wrote: "The results indicate that there is a relationship, even in a single country, between dairy product consumption and the incidence of IDDM that is confined to fluid milk consumption."[11]

One interesting study conducted in Finland showed that an increased diabetes risk exists for infants who were given cow's milk even

Diabetes Care 1994;17(1):13

Early cow milk exposure may increase juvenile diabetes risk by about 1.5 times.

QUOTE

"Diabetes does not occur in diabetes-prone rodents reared on a diet free of cow's milk for the first two to three months of life, indicating that cow's milk protein can trigger the disease."

New England Journal of Medicine 1992;327(5):302-307

though they were also being breast-fed. Breast-feeding did not provide any apparent protective effect in the presence of cow's milk.[12]

Nature vs Nurture

As a result of such findings, researchers are beginning to view environmental factors as being as important as those of heredity in the development of this type of diabetes. In the debate of "nature versus nurture," it seems that "nurture" is becoming increasingly important.

Studies with identical twins have shown that for every three sets of twins genetically prone to IDDM, in only one set did both twins develop the disease.[13] While such discoveries are not conculsive, they do show that environmental factors may be as important as heredity ones in contracting IDDM.

Letters printed in one journal suggested that adult onset, or type II, diabetes may be promoted by the combination of fat, sugar, and

(Continued on p. 20)

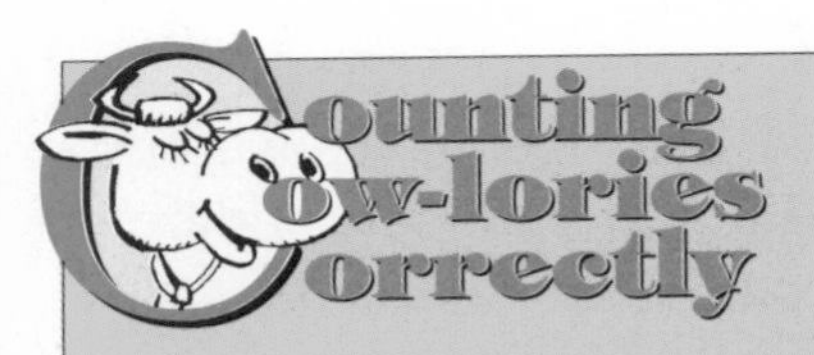

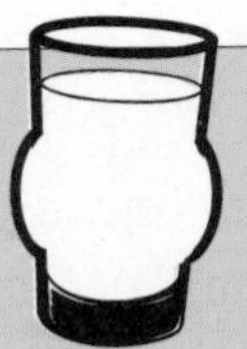

The carton says whole milk is 3.5% fat. Sounds good! But that's 3.5% fat by WEIGHT! How many of milk's cow-lories come from fat? Add it up for yourself:

Serving Size	**8 ounces**
Calories per serving	**160**
Fat per serving	**9 grams**
9 gm fat x 9 cal/gm*	**81 calories**

* Fat always contains 9 calories per gram

Simple math reveals that more than 50% (81 of 160 calories) of milk's cow-lories come from fat—and that's udderly too high! Don't be fooled by skewed statistics.

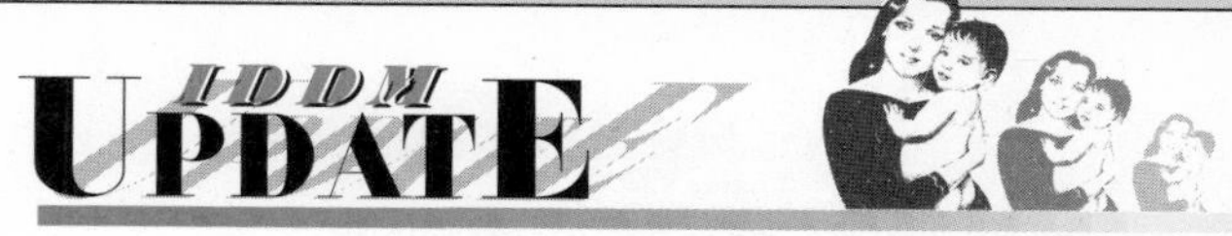

More reports on the possible milk/IDDM link

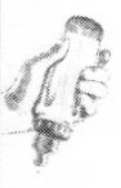

"Ecological and time-series studies consistently showed a relationship between type I diabetes and either cow's milk exposure or diminished breast-feeding."

Diabetes Care 1994;17(1):13-19

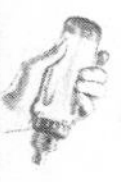

"Epidemiologic and serologic data in humans also suggest a relation between cow's milk and diabetes."

New England Journal of Medicine 1992;327(5):302-307

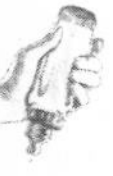

"In the largest population studied thus far, we showed that introduction of dairy products during early infancy, but not duration of breast-feeding, was associated with an increased risk of IDDM."

"In several countries, a high positive correlation was found between the per capita consumption of dairy products and the risk of IDDM."

Diabetes 1993;42:1786-1789

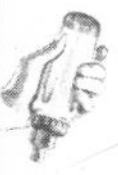

"(Cow's milk protein) may play a fundamental role in the development of...IDDM."

Diabetes 1996;45(2):178-182

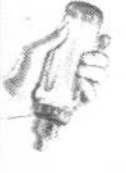

"We infer that the proteins of cow's milk may trigger the autoimmune process of IDDM."

Diabetes Care 1993;16(7):984-989

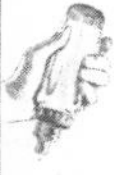

"Bovine serum albumin (protein) detected in infant formula is a possible trigger for IDDM."

J American Dietetic Association 1994;94(3):314-316

milk in the diet.[14] In clinical studies, such a combination has been shown to cause hyperglycemia[14], obesity,[15] and rapid growth.[15]

Years ago, mothers were warned not to feed their infants evaporated milk because of its high levels of sugar and cow's protein. Perhaps these dietary elements, coupled with our consumption of other high-fat, high-protein animal products, could be a factor in the proliferation of adult-onset (non-insulin dependent) diabetes, which has increased more than 700 percent among 45 to 54-year-olds in the United States since World War II![16]

Something to Sneeze At?

Could dairy products have a link to the runny noses and itchy eyes of allergy sufferers? Allergic reactions to milk can appear in unusual ways, including constipation, eczema,

I have run into patients who undergo marked alterations in behavior patterns when ingesting dairy products, and whose behavior is totally changed by withholding them.

John J. Murray, MD, (pediatrician)
Letter, Pediatrics 1979;64(5):699

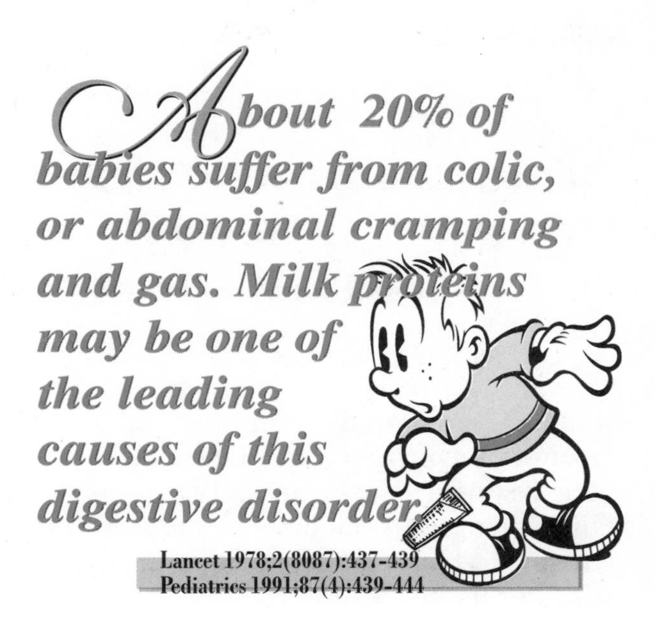

dermatitis, vomiting, headaches, psychological problems, retarded growth, and fatigue.[17]

Even bed-wetting has been tied to dairy products.[18] Food sensitivities, which can lead to allergies, can develop in infants as a result of the absorption of incompletely digested animal protein.[19]

Since milk allergy in adults is common and may be misdiagnosed as a different allergy,[20] the milk/allergy connection deserves further research.

An estimated 50 million Americans experience intestinal discomfort after consuming dairy products. Symptoms include bloating, stomach pain, cramps, gas, or diarrhea.

Postgraduate Medicine 1994;95(1):113-120

One recent study found that infants fed casein-rich evaporated milk developed a metabolic disorder called transient tyrosinemia (a failure to properly metabolize the amino acid tyrosine) which resulted in learning disabilities later in life.[21]

Intolerable!

Allergies to cow's milk are more common than many realize. One may be sensitive to milk protein, or to lactose (milk sugar), or to both,[22] or to drug residues in the milk.

Lactose intolerant people cannot digest this milk sugar because they lack a digestive enzyme known as lactase. Lactose intolerance is a common problem encountered in clinical practice,[23] with as many as 90 percent of Asians and Blacks having the disorder worldwide.[23]

A recent three-year study of 129 children suffering from recurrent abdominal pain, gas, bloating, diarrhea and constipation found that 25% were lactose intolerant.[24] When they were given a lactose-free diet, many of the symptoms disappeared.[24] According to the researchers, 15 percent of school-aged children have recurrent stomach pain.[24]

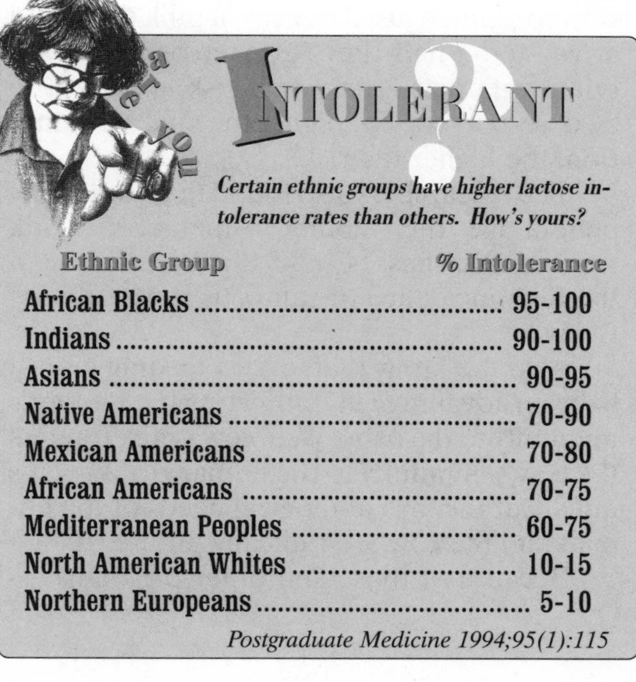

are you INTOLERANT?

Certain ethnic groups have higher lactose intolerance rates than others. How's yours?

Ethnic Group	% Intolerance
African Blacks	95-100
Indians	90-100
Asians	90-95
Native Americans	70-90
Mexican Americans	70-80
African Americans	70-75
Mediterranean Peoples	60-75
North American Whites	10-15
Northern Europeans	5-10

Postgraduate Medicine 1994;95(1):115

Cow's Milk and Cataracts

Some researchers even point to milk drinking and lactose intolerance as being involved in the development of senile (age-related) cataracts,[25] although more evidence is needed.

According to the research, if a person's digestive system has problems digesting lactose (and galactose, a component of lactose), damage to the lens of the eye may be a result.

Individuals with lactose malabsorption who consumed just 3 ounces of milk daily, had a two-and-a-half times greater risk of developing cataracts.[25] And that risk appeared to be dose-related: The higher the milk consumption, the higher the risk.

The researchers also found that as healthy people age, their ability to metabolize milk sugar diminishes.[25] Could this be a factor in the high incidence of cataracts in the elderly today?

Also, we know that breast feeding gives a baby an advantage in tranferring the mother's immunity to the baby. Well, cow's milk tranfers the cow's immunity to the human drinking it's milk. But the immunological needs of the human and the cow are radically different!

Because of these and other problems as-

“QUOTE”

Adults who consume large quantities of milk, who have high lactase activity,...suffer repeated small galactose challenges, accumulation of galactitol in the lens, and a greater likelihood of developing senile cataracts.

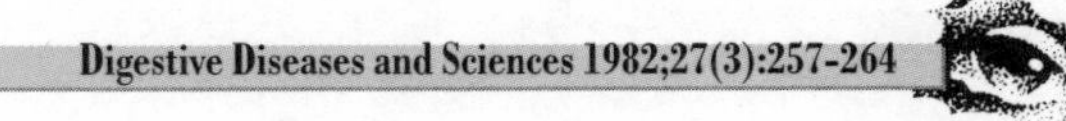

Digestive Diseases and Sciences 1982;27(3):257-264

sociated with cow's milk consumption in infancy, many pediatricians are recommending soy-based formulas for infants whose mothers are unable to nurse. Compared to casein-based formulas, soy formulas are more easily digested, although allergies can develop with soy milk formulas in sensitive infants.[1]

Infants and children are the not the only ones at risk, however. Dairy products tend to be high in fat, and that can increase one's risk of heart disease.[26] While there are questions about the milk-heart disease link, surprising new studies show stronger correlations of death from ischemic heart disease (low blood

Milk fat has been identified as a (cholesterol- elevating) fat because it contains cholesterol and is primarily saturated.

Journal of Dairy Science 1991;74(11):4002-4012

supply to the heart which can cause chest pain or even heart attack) with nonfat dairy products than with dairy fat or margarine![27] What could be causing this surprising action?

The Rise and Fall...

It may be caused by a protein link that is most fascinating. Simply put, nutrient utilization in the cells of the body depends upon the balanced working of two hormones, insulin and glucagon. Insulin's job is to put what you eat into your cells, and glucagon's job is to take it out.

The casein in milk, as well as other animal protein, causes a higher level of insulin secretion and a lower level of glucagon secretion in the human body. Plant proteins, however, do not seem to have the same effect.

The higher content of branched chain amino acids (valine, isoleucine, and leucine) in animal products appears to cause this rise in insulin and drop in glucagon.[28]A high insulin level, among other things, causes the human body to become very efficient at taking the carboyhrates one eats and turn them into fats, especially cholesterol![28]

The Lactose—Link

Although casein, through the animal protein effect described above, is able to elevate cholesterol levels, lactose is a likely culprit. Milk is high in lactose, whether it is whole milk, low-fat, or skim. Butter is low in lactose, but is about 85 percent fat. Specific national and eth-

"Any time a patient of mine is found to have streptococcal pharyngitis or pyoderma, we can establish by history that he has ingested milk protein within five days..."

Frank Oski, MD (pediatrician)
Don't Drink Your Milk, p. 24

“QUOTE”

Milk and many components of milk (butterfat, milk protein, calcium from milk, and riboflavin)... were positively related to coronary heart disease mortality for all 40 countries studied.

Circulation 1993;88(6):2771-2779

nic data, as well as studies done in other countries, suggest that a low-lactose diet is more protective against ischemic heart disease than even a diet high in fiber![27]

It's Fat, And That's That?

Even with all the emphasis on excess fat in the diet today, many Americans are still unaware of the fact that most of the fat they eat is *hidden* in their food. (See chart on page 31.) Most dietary fat comes from meat, cheese, cream, and milk.[29] While red meat is our largest source of fat calories, we “herd up” quite a number from dairy products, too.[29]

The high cholesterol and triglyceride levels that milk can cause are both associated with higher risk of coronary heart disease. Indeed, studies have shown that adult milk drinkers do tend to have elevated levels of both cholesterol and triglycerides.[30] Because of this, many today feel that switching to low-fat or skim milk will take care of the problem. But such a switch may cause even bigger problems!

It's true that low-fat or skim milk products will reduce one's saturated fat intake, and thus could help lower his or her blood cholesterol levels. But remember, these lower-fat dairy products still contain about the same levels of casein and lactose, which, as we have seen, appear to be a factor in America's number one killer disease, heart disease.

Milk's fat, casein, and lactose are not the

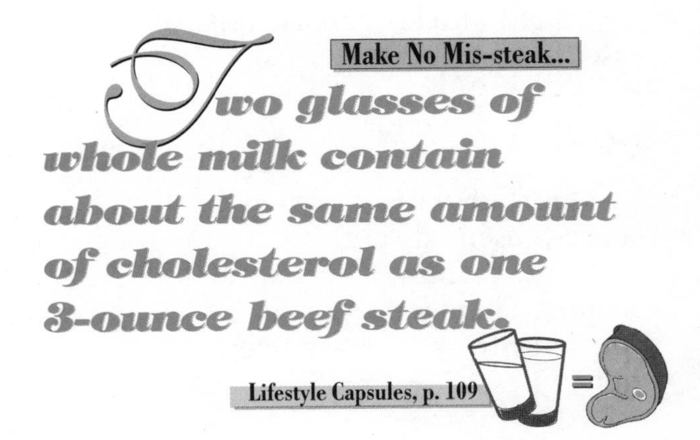

Lifestyle Capsules, p. 109

Greenland Eskimos, who have a very low incidence of ischemic heart disease, have a high-fat, high-protein diet, but a very low intake of milk.

British J of Preventive and Social Medicine 1977;31:81-85

only things to consider when it comes to your heart's health. Some researchers are reporting that lactalbumin, another animal protein in milk, may also be tied to heart disease.[31]

In addition, problems associated with heating milk proteins during the pasteurization process, and the tendency to consume too many calories on a dairy-based diet, are also associated with an increased risk of heart disease.[32]

2 Glasses A Day?

One study author concluded that "The evidence presented (in this study) suggests that milk intake may be harmful to coronary health....There is no justification for the campaign to drink at least one pint (2 cups) daily."[32]

(Continued on p. 32)

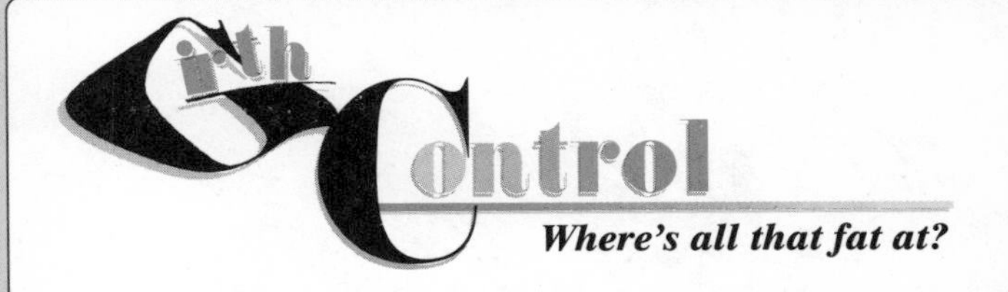

Where's all that fat at?

If you're tired of playing the "hide-and-seek" fat game, this chart is for you!

Fat Content of Foods

Food	% Calories/Fat
Cream cheese	90
Beef, pork	65-83
Pasteurized, processed cheese	60-85
Ice Cream	55
Milk, whole	50
Cottage Cheese	36
Grains	5-15
Legumes	5-10
Milk, skim	2
Fruits, vegetables	1-5

***To Your Health*, p. 196.**

One quart of whole milk per day adds 35 grams of fat to your diet. Couple that with the other "hidden" and visible fat eaten daily, and you can see why milk adds to our "growing" problem in the United States today!

Osteoporosis is caused by a number of things, one of the most important things being *too much* dietary protein!

American Journal of Clinical Nutrition 1974;27(9):916-925
Journal of Nutrition 1981;111(3):545-552; 553-562
Science 1986;233(4763):519-520

One final point here. Research has shown that adult milk drinkers who drink a large amount of milk daily (more than 200 ml—a large glass), have higher total cholesterol levels, higher low-density lipoprotein-cholesterol ("bad" cholesterol) levels, and higher triglyceride levels than those who drink less than 60 ml per day.[30]

Those who consumed large amounts of milk also had more problems with obesity than those who consumed less milk.[30]

Dairy calories are very concentrated, as the chart on page 31 shows, which is one reason why people who consume dairy products frequently could have weight control problems.

What About My Cow-cium?

At this point some may be asking, "But milk is the ideal source of calcium. And where can I get a better protein than from milk?"

Those are excellent, important questions, so let's briefly address them here. (For a more in-depth look at protein and human protein needs, you can purchase the ***Let's Eat*** video

Enough Is *Enough!*

*Just how much calcium do we **really** need?*

Calcium Need in Milligrams:

***World intake** (most populations)* **300-500**
World Health Org. minimum **400-500**
US Food/Nutrition Board **800**
NIH recommendation **1,000-1,500**

McDougall's Medicine, p. 67

(NOTE: Actual calcium needs vary with age, amount of exercise, dietary habits, available sunlight, and other factors. Many experts agree that someone on a low-protein diet who gets regular, weight-bearing exercise in fresh air and sunlight, would have much lower daily calcium needs (perhaps 400-800 mg) than someone on a meat-based diet with little or no exercise or activity outside (perhaps as high as 1,200 mg or more).

One tasty way to get your daily calcium supply is to eat 1-2 cups (cooked volume) of dark greens like collards, mustards, kale, etc.

(See chart, page 51.) *Milton Crane, MD*

and book entitled *High Protein: Giving Your Bones a Break*. You can purchase them at many book stores, or by calling 1-800-453-8732.)

Boning Up On The Facts

In the United States, approximately 15-20 million people have osteoporosis.[33] Osteoporosis is a disease caused in part by the loss of bone calcium which results in very weak, brittle bones.

People with osteoporosis can experience low-impact fractures—fractures caused by minor accidents that normally would not damage a bone. They can even have spontaneous fractures—a hip may fracture while they're getting up out of a chair, for example.

Dietary protein increases production of acid (in the blood) which can be neutralized by calcium mobilized from the skeleton.

American Journal of Clinical Nutrition 1995;61(4):909

About 50,000 Americans die each year of problems related in some way to osteoporosis.

Osteoporosis International 1993;3(3):148-153

Osteoporosis occurs most frequently in affluent Western societies. Its care and treatment costs $4 billion each year in the United States alone.[34]

In countries where little or no meat or dairy products are consumed, there is actually far less osteoporosis than in the United States.[35] In fact, studies have shown that dairy products are not necessarily protective against developing osteoporosis.[36]

It should be no surprise, then, that in spite of our high intake of calcium-rich dairy products, osteoporosis causes 1.3 million fractures in people 45 years and older each year in the United States.[34,37]

Because these facts are opposite of what

we have been taught, let's review them again just for clarity. In third world countries where milk is not regularly consumed, osteoporosis is rare. Contrary to what many of us have been taught, osteoporosis is most common in countries where the largest amount of dairy products are consumed.[38]

How is it that our high intake of dairy products, which is supposed to protect against osteoporosis, is not yielding better results for those who consume large amounts dairy products? There are several possible reasons.

Protein's Bare Bones Action

First, while daily calcium intake is important, numerous studies have clearly demonstrated that *too much dietary protein, not too little calcium*, is a major cause of osteoporosis.[39] Why?

Too much protein causes an excess of hydrogen ions in the blood, which elevates blood acid levels. Because high acid levels can be dangerous, the body "buffers," or neutralizes the blood acid levels by drawing calcium from the bones. The resulting waste products, including the calcium, are excreted in the urine.[39]

Dr. T. Colin Campbell, a researcher and professor of nutritional biochemistry at Cornell University in New York, explains it this way:

"When the body metabolizes more of these (animal) proteins than it needs, sulfur-based acids are produced. To neutralize these acids, the body draws on its stores of calcium. Instead of being used to build bone, the calcium spills into the urine."[40]

A study conducted at the Institute of Child

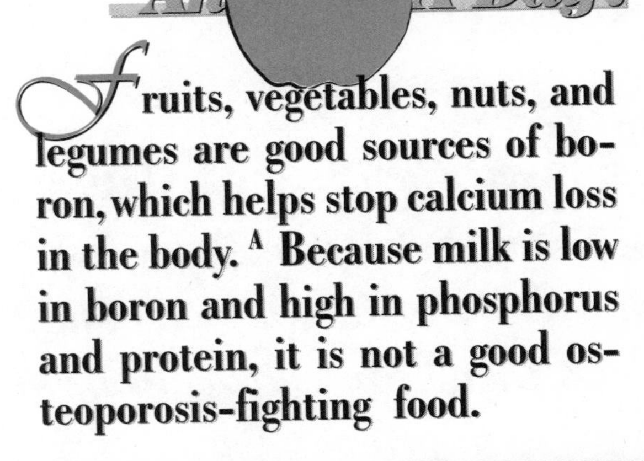

Fruits, vegetables, nuts, and legumes are good sources of boron, which helps stop calcium loss in the body.[A] Because milk is low in boron and high in phosphorus and protein, it is not a good osteoporosis-fighting food.

A. *Dr. Forrest H. Nielsen,* USDA, in ***Nutiriton Today*** **Jan/Feb 1988;4-7**
FSAEB Journal **1987;1:394-397**

Nutrition in Dortmund, Germany, seems to confirm Dr. Campbell's statement. In that study, researcers found that when subjects switched from a lacto-ovo vegetarian diet to one that included more animal protein, acid levels went up—and so did their calcium loss![40] They also reported that the higher the animal protein levels, the more dramatic the calcium loss became.[41]

The Breaking News

In another investigation, researchers studying 85,180 women over a 10-year period, found that excess dietary protein did, indeed, in-

(Continued on p. 40)

Even when eating 1,400 mg of calcium daily, one can lose up to 4% of his or her bone mass each year while consuming a high-protein diet.

American Journal of Clinical Nutrition 1979;32(4):741-749

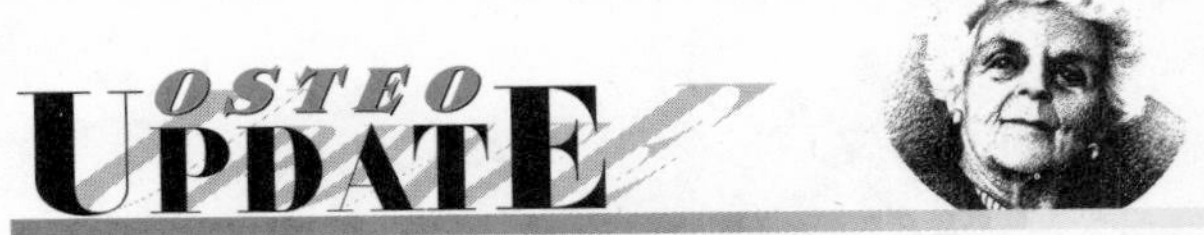

More on the animal protein/osteoporosis link

Excessive protein intake could account for the 1.0% to 1.5% loss in bone mass each year typically seen in postmenopausal women.

● J of Laboratory and Clinical Medicine 1982;99(1):46-55

Methionine (a sulfur amino acid) intake in humans resulted in increased urinary calcium excretion.

● American J of Clincial Nutrition 1994;59(6):1356-1361

Sulfur amino acids in animal products seem to be primarily responsible for the increased calcium loss.

● Calcified Tissue International 1989;44(5):335-338

Meat-based diets are more acid producing than lacto-ovo vegetarian (LOV) diets; and LOV diets are more acid producing than vegan diets.

● J of the American Dietetic Association 1985;85(7):841-845

Increasing protein intake by 50 grams caused an extra 60 mg of calcium to be excreted in the urine.

● Journal of Nutrition 1990;120(1):134-136

In Western countries, eating more than 75 g/day of protein is likely to cause excessive calcium loss.

● J of Bone and Joint Surgery (Am) 1967;49(5):915-924

Study subjects had a negative calcium balance eating 142 g/day of protein and 1,400 mg/day of calcium: a positive calcium balance resulted when subjects got 50 g/day of protein and 500 mg of calcium.*

● Federation Proceedings 1981;40(9):2429-2433

* Negative calcium balance = bones are being robbed of calcium
Positive calcium balance = calcium available for bone maintenance

Under controlled conditions the level of dietary protein has a profound and sustained effect on urinary calcium (levels)...

Federation Proceedings 1981;40(9):2429-2433

crease their forearm fracture rates due to low-trauma circumstances.[42]

In the study, women consuming 95 or more grams of protein daily had an age-adjusted increased forearm-fracture risk of 1.23 times, compared to women who consumed less than 68 grams per day.[42]

The researchers also found that for women who consumed higher amounts of animal protein during both their adult and teenage years, the risk of forearm fracture was "significantly increased by 44%."[42]

Such increases in fracture rates were observed for protein derived from animal sources but no increased risk was found with higher consumption of vegetable protein.[42]

Even consuming 90 grams of soy protein a day did not cause bone calcium loss in one study.[43] Such a high level of animal protein intake, however, has been shown to cause a definite and measurable calcium loss.

Based on the conclusions of these and other studies, Americans may, in fact, be too worried about getting enough protein. But how did such over-concern about protein originate?

Are You "Over-Proteinized?

Early estimates of infant protein needs were greatly exaggerated. Between 1948 and 1974, protein estimates decreased by about two-thirds, from more than 3 grams per kilogram (g/kg) of body weight to just a little over 1 g/kg of body weight.[44]

Compounding the protein concern problem was the fact that for years many experts

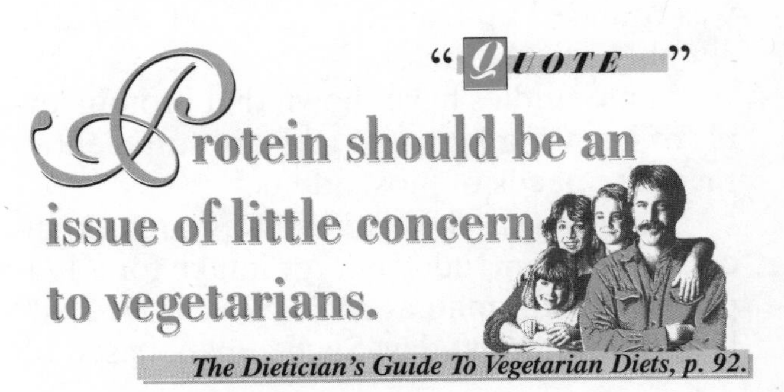

Dairy products may play a major role in the development of allergies, asthma, sleep difficulties, and migraine headaches.

Israel Journal of Medical Sciences 1983;19(9):806-809
Pediatrics 1989;84(4):595-603

viewed plant proteins as being somehow inferior in quality to animal proteins.

Now, however, it is widely established that eating two plant proteins at the same meal, or at two different meals in the same day, will promote more growth than eating a single animal protein.[45]

Today, the recommended daily allowance (RDA) of protein for adults is just 0.8 g/kg of body weight[46]—and that includes a very generous built-in safety margin of 25% to account for individual variation. In addition, the RDA was rounded up from 0.75 g/kg to 0.8 g/kg to simplify calculations.

Some studies have shown that protein levels of just 0.5 g/kg to 0.6 g/kg are sufficient to meet the needs of most adults.[47]

According to the National Research Council, the recommended energy intake for a 174-pound (79 kg) man aged 25-50 years is 2,900 kcal (kilocalories)/day. Such a man, based on

(Continued on p. 44)

It's All in the Numbers!

Can a plant-based diet supply the 9-10% protein we need in our daily caloric intake? A quick look shows that the answer is all in the numbers!

Food/Serving Size	Protein (%)	Protein (g)
Brown rice (1 cup)	8.5	4.9
White rice (1 cup)	7.4	4.1
Barley, pearled (1 cup)	9.4	16.4
Garbanzo beans (1 cup)	21.6	14.5
Lentils (1 cup)	31.0	17.9
Lima beans (1 cup)	27.1	14.7
Tofu, raw (1/2 cup)	42.5	10.0
Soy milk (1 cup)	33.4	6.6
Peanuts, dried (1 oz.)	18.1	7.3
Broccoli, raw (1/2 cup)	43.3	1.3
Carrots, raw (1 med.)	9.0	0.7
Whl. wht. bread (1 sl.)	15.7	2.4
Grn. beans, boiled (1 cup)	21.8	1.2
Apple, raw w/skin (med.)	1.5	0.3
Banana, raw (med.)	4.6	1.2
Bagel (1)	14.7	6.0

Source: *Bowes and Church's Food Values of Portions Commonly Used*, 16th edition, 1994.

NOTE: While protein derived from a mix of the above foods is sufficient to meet daily protein needs, it will not exert the same calcium-leaching effect on the bones that a high intake of animal protein will.

the RDA requirements for protein, would need just 63.2 grams per day (0.8 g/kg x 79 kg). That would account for less than 9% of his total recommended caloric intake each day.

By looking at the chart on page 43, it is obvious that a vegetarian would have no problem at all meeting that need!

Recent surveys of Americans show that between 14% and 18% of their calories come from protein (about 110 grams per day),[48] far more than the recommended daily allowance (RDA)! And the major source of that protein is animal products. The higher the intake of animal protein, the more calcium is leached from the bones.

More On Boron

Another reason why America's high intake of dairy products is not protecting against osteoporosis is that milk, meat, and eggs are poor sources of boron.

Boron may be important in preventing osteoporosis because it helps stop the loss of calcium from the body and may play a role in adjusting the level of estrogen, which, in turn, affects bone metabolism.[49] Where can you find boron? Good sources include leafy green vegetables, fruits, grains, and nuts.

The Acid Test

Compounding American's excess protein problem is the fact that animal protein differs in both content and composition from vegetable protein.

Proteins are made up of various combi-

Increasing one's protein intake by 100% may cause calcium loss to double.*

Journal of Nutrition 1981;111(3):553-562

NOTE: *Such a statement is very important because the average American consumes about twice as much protein as his or her body needs!*

nations of about 20 different building blocks called amino acids. Two of these twenty amino acids, methionine and cysteine, contain sulfur.

In the body, sulfur is is oxidized, or changed, to sulfate and then linked with calcium to form calcium sulfate which is excreted by the kidneys. Obviously, this whole process imposes a calcium-losing effect on the bones,[50] which can lead to osteoporosis.

Packing A Protein Punch!

Animal foods usually contain about 3 times more protein than plant foods and are relatively high in sulfur. Roughly twice as much methionine is present in meat as in grains, and

(Continued on p. 48)

The first study showing that animal protein could cause calcium loss was published in 1930[A]! Why is it that almost 70 years later many people still don't know that?

A: Journal of Biological Chemistry 1930;87:669

Have You Heard the INCOMPLETE STORY?

Have you heard the incomplete protein claim? It says that plant proteins are incomplete proteins, so you have to combine different ones at each meal in order to get a complete, beneficial protein? Is such a claim true? Is food combining necessary?

"Plant sources of protein alone can provide adequate amounts of the essential and nonessential amino acids, assuming that dietary protein sources from plants are reasonably varied and that caloric intake is sufficient to meet energy needs....Conscious combining of these foods within a given meal as the complementary protein dictum suggests is unnecessary."

J of the American Dietetic Association 1993;93(11):1317-1319

five times more is present in meat than in beans.[51,52]

Even though the relative sulfur amino acid content of grains is similar to that of most animal foods, research suggests that plant foods, in general, are less likely to cause urinary calcium excretion.[53]

For the most part, meat-based diets are more acid producing than plant-based diets.[54] Not surprisingly, lacto-ovo vegetarian diets are more acid producing than vegan diets.[54] Hence, diets containing animal foods will tend to cause more calcium loss and a greater osteoporosis risk.

No Bones About It!

Generally, for every excess gram of protein consumed, calcium loss increases by about 1 mg.[55] One study reported that increasing animal protein consumption caused a fivefold increase in blood acid levels![55] And that means calcium loss from the bones and teeth.

Interestingly, in 34 cross-cultural studies done in 16 countries, eating animal protein was linked to increased hip fracture rates in humans.[56]

In 1972, author Frances Moore Lappe claimed that animal foods are a superior protein, while plant foods are inferior. If eating plant proteins, she wrote, a complicated method of combining "complementary protein" foods had to be followed. Ten years later, she realized her error and wrote:

"In combatting the myth that meat is the only way to get high-quality protein, I reinforced another myth. I gave the impression that in order to get enough protein without meats, considerable care was needed in choosing foods."

Nutrition Action Newsletter, October 1982, p. 10

One's dietary calcium-to-protein ratio may be the best predictor of bone health and may be more important than total calcium intake.[57] A lower total protein intake will probably reduce calcium requirement and promote bone health.

Even though bones may lose calcium with high blood-acid levels, the body does not replace it by absorbing higher levels of calcium from new food intake.[58] So, as long as protein intake is high, bone calcium levels suffer as

Greens such as kale, broccoli, and bok choy are as good as milk in terms of their calcium absorbability.

Environmental Nutrition, January 1994, p. 3
The American Journal of Clinical Nutrition 1990;51:656-657

calcium is robbed from them in order to maintain a proper balance elsewhere.

The Incomplete Story

This may be shocking to those who always thought that animal proteins were *complete* proteins, and thus superior to plant proteins. The truth is, all plant proteins are complete proteins because they provide all the essential amino acids needed for maintaining good health.[52,59] They also tend to be somewhat lower in sulfur-containing amino acids.[60]

Throughout the world, protein deficiency is usually the result of an inadequate caloric intake (calorie deficiency), and not consumption of poor-quality protein.[61]

Protein is abundant in grains, vegetables, beans, and nuts, but tends to be less concentrated than in animal products. The most wholesome diet will contain a daily variety of plant protein sources like beans, grains, vegetables, fruits, and nuts.

The ability of plant protein alone to meet protein needs was demonstrated in the Michigan State University Bread Study.[62] For 50 days, university students, aged 19 to 27, ate diets that provided 70 g of protein daily, 90%

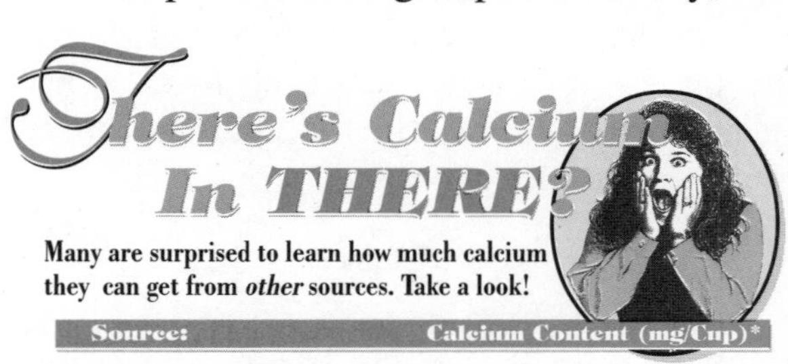

Source	Calcium Content (mg/Cup)*
Roasted almonds	369
Soy flour (defatted)	366
Garbanzo beans (dry)	300
Cow's milk	291
Mustard greens, cooked	284
Soy milk (calcium fortified)	240
Collards, cooked	220
Kale, cooked	206
Broccoli, cooked	136
Raisins (packed)	102

* Refer again to the chart on p. VI in the foreword of this book.

Nutrition Almanac, McGraw Hill, pages 200-230
Product package nutrition information

to 95% of which came from the wheat flour in their bread.[62] The other 5% to 10% of their protein came from fruits and vegetables.[62] They didn't consume any animal protein.

Test results showed that, on average, subjects had a proper nitrogen balance, revealing adequate protein intake.[62]

Nitrogen balance is also maintained in countries where rice is a staple food, supplying as much as 75% of the daily caloric intake.[63]

Cow-cium Cow-nts!

Fourth, the high casein content of milk may inhibit calcium absorption.[1] Some studies have shown that the high calcium content of milk

The average man in the US eats 175% more protein than the recommended daily allowance (RDA) and the average woman eats 144% more!

Surgeon General's Report on Nutrition and Health, 1988, p. 69

"QUOTE"

These data suggest that during adult life, a reduction in dietary intake of fat and proteins of animal origin may contribute to a substantial reduction in the incidence of breast cancer...in population subgroups with high intake of animal products.

Journal of National Cancer Institute 1989;81(4):278-286

may inhibit iron absorption also.[64] According to one report, calcium absorption is higher from eating certain greens than from drinking milk![65]

All green vegetables contain calcium because it is an essential element in photosynthesis, the process by which plants convert sunlight into energy. Generally, the darker green the plant, the more calcium it contains. Most grains, beans, nuts, and many fruits also con-

Nations with the highest dietary fat consumption also have the highest rates of prostate and breast cancer.

Advances in Cancer Research 1980;32:237-345
Cancer Research 1975;35(11 Pt. 2):3374-3383

tain calcium. Fortified orange juice is also a tasty, refreshing calcium source.

The Cancer Connection

While the evidence linking milk to an increased osteoporosis risk is increasing, what about cancer? Could the high-protein and high-fat levels found in milk and other dairy products be contributing to the growing cancer crisis we are seeing in the United States today?

A report from the National Academy of Sciences states: "Evidence from both epidemiological and laboratory studies suggest that high protein intake may be associated with an increased risk of cancers at certain sites."[66]

This should be expected since, as pointed out earlier, animal protein consumption causes higher secretions of insulin in the body.

Research has shown that cancer cells are dependent upon insulin for growth.[67]

An Italian study revealed that women consuming a diet rich in saturated fat and animal protein had a significanly increased risk of breast cancer when compared to women with low intakes of saturated fat and protein.[68]

Could it be that the saturated fat was the cause, and not the protein? Perhaps, but both animal studies[69] and ecologic data[70] have shown that protein intake alone may be positively related to an increased breast cancer risk.

While more research is needed on the milk-cancer link, animal protein consumption has been linked to increased colon cancer risk.[71]

"QUOTE"

Dietary factors (mainly high fat and animal protein intake) appear to be the most important risk determinants for colon cancer.

Regulatory Toxicology and Pharmacology 1986;6(1):24-54

As a group, control patients (in a cancer study) were more likely to report never drinking whole milk; cancer patients more often reported frequent consumption of whole milk.

Nutrition and Cancer 1990;13(1-2):89-99

Several studies have associated eating animal protein with both non-Hodgkin's lymphoma[72,73] and Hodgkin's disease.[73] Several other studies have specifically linked milk consumption with non-Hodgkin's lymphoma.[74]

A "SIGNIFICANT RISK"

In a study involving 3,334 cancer patients, frequent whole milk consumption led to "significant risk increases for cancers of the oral cavity, stomach, rectum, lung, and breast."[75]

Milk's high fat content was considered to be a large factor, but did not completely explain the overall increase in risk.[75]

In a separate study of 569 lung cancer patients, consumption of whole milk three or more times daily was associated with a two-

(Continued on p. 58)

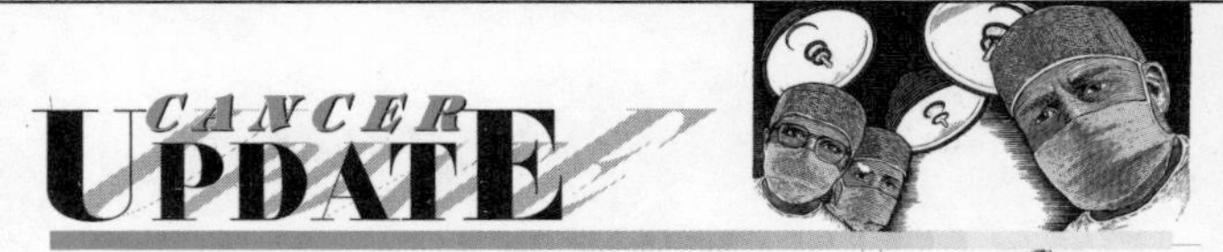

More on the dairy/cancer connection

There is much controversy surrounding the possibility of a connection between milk and various cancers. While some studies report that milk intake reduces the risk of certain cancers, other studies disagree. Here is a sampling of some of those studies.

- **One reason to suspect that whole milk increases the risk of lung cancer is that milk is the 4th leading source of calories and the second leading source of saturated fat in the typical American diet.**

  - International Journal of Cancer 1989;43:608-611

- **Animal fat, cholesterol, and saturated fat were positively correlated with pancreatic cancer mortality.**

  - Revista de Sanidad e Higiene Publica 1994;68(3):361-376

- **A "significant dose-response relationship" was found between animal fat intake and ovarian cancer risk.**

  - British Journal of Cancer 1989;59(1):92-96

- **Galactose metabolism differs between women with and without a family history of ovarian cancer, suggesting that it may be a genetic risk factor for ovarian cancer.**

  - Cancer 1994;74(4):1309-1317

- **Whole milk is a leading source of cholesterol in the U.S. diet and dietary cholesterol has been associated with cancers of the breast, lung, and colon.**

  - American Journal of Clinical Nutrition 1983;37(2):192-193
  - American Journal of Epidemiology 1987;125(3):351-363
  - Broitman, S. Dietary Fat and Cancer. Progress in Clinical and Biological Research, 1986;222:435-459
  - International Journal of Cancer 1989;43:608-611

Note: Milk offers no nutritional benefit that cannot be attained from other sources, so why use it and take a possible risk?

"QUOTE"

The subclasses of casein, amino acid sequence, and profiles of human and bovine milk differ markedly.

Proceedings of the Society for Experimental Biology and Medicine 1990 Nov, p. 143.

fold increase in lung cancer risk, compared to those who never consumed milk.[76]

In a 20-year study done in Spain, researchers found a positive link between milk and cheese consumption and pancreatic cancer in males.[77] Eating eggs increased the pancreatic cancer risk in females.[77] Fruit consumption seemed to result in reduced cancer risk.[77]

A "SIGNIFICANT TREND"

Surprisingly, some studies have revealed "a highly significant trend"[78] linking increased ovarian cancer risk to galactose, a component of lactose.[78] Researchers found that women with ovarian cancer used more yogurt and cottage cheese, both high in galactose, than did those in the control groups.[78]

The milk sugar in these products is prehydrolyzed, and it appears that this form of lactose increases galactose levels and may encourage increased ovarian tumor formation.

If their findings are confirmed, "avoidance of lactose-rich foods by adults may be a way of primary prevention of ovarian cancer."[79]

While some researchers question the lactose-ovarian cancer link, science has generally confirmed that animal fat, including the high fat content of whole milk, may lead to an in-

Studies show that the milk sugar lactose may aid in mineral absorption, and that includes one element no one wants—lead. Weanling rats given normal doses of lactose had increased levels of lead in their tissues. As lactose levels were increased, lead levels increased also. Even moderately elevated lead concentrations in tissues have been linked to learning disabilities and other serious problems in children and adults.

Science 1981;211(4477):61-63
Journal of Learning Disabilities 1994;27(6):393-399
Environmental Research 1993;60(1):30-43
International Journal of Epidemiology 1993;22(5):891-897

creased incidence of ovarian and other cancers.[68,80] But in the study cited above,[78] the incidence of ovarian cancer was not linked to the fat or protein in the dairy products, but to the milk sugar, galactose.[78]

TELLING "D" TRUTH

Most people who drink milk haven't heard of its possible cancer connection, and usually drink it for several reasons:

1. To get calcium for strong bones,
2. To get enough dietary protein,
3. To get vitamin D.

Our discussion has addressed those first two concerns, but we must talk about vitamin D before moving on.

The primary job of vitamin D is helping the body maintain proper calcium levels in the blood.

Exposure to sunlight provides most humans with their vitamin D requirement.

Journal of Nutrition 1996;126(4 Suppl):1159S-1164S

Just D Facts...

Milk may not be a reliable source of vitamin D because some samples have had 500 times too much[A] (which can be toxic[B]) while other samples have had little or none at all[C]!

A: New England Journal of Medicine 1992;326:1173-1177
B: The Dietician's Guide to Vegetarian Diets, p. 180
C: Journal of Nutrition 1996;126(4 Suppl):1159S-1164S

While the current RDA for vitamin D in adults is a very generous 5.0 micrograms,[81] the average daily intake for adults in the United States is between 1.25 and 1.75 micrograms.[81]

The difference between the RDA and actual intake is probably made up by sunlight's ability to stimulate the body to make vitamin D, especially during summer months. Adults need 10 to 15 minutes of sunlight two or three times a week during the summer to ensure proper vitamin D levels.[82]

While senior citizens and dark-skinned people require longer sun exposure to meet vitamin D needs, some feel that even brief exposure to sunlight is the same as ingesting 5.0 micrograms of vitamin D.[83]

Unfortunately, many senior citizens are apparently not able to adequately convert cholesterol in the skin to the precursor moloecule that later becomes active vitamin D.[84] For them, an adequate source of vitamin D must be utilized to lower osteoporosis risk.[84]

Toxici-D

Vitamin D is not present in any plant foods, and is supplied poorly in fortified foods. Such fortification must be closely monitored because too much vitamin D can be toxic, especially in young children. Toxic levels can cause excessive calcium levels in the blood and urine, which can lead to calcium deposits in soft tissue and irreversible kidney and heart damage.

Vitamin D increases aluminum absorption, and high aluminum levels in the body may cause an Alzheimer's-like disease.[85]

According to federal regulations, one quart of milk should contain 400 IU (10 micrograms) of vitamin D.[86] Consuming as little as 45 micrograms of vitamin D_3 in young children has

"QUOTE"

"Bovine leukemia virus is leukemogenic (can cause leukemia) in at least two mammalian species, is wide-spread in commercial dairy herds, and can infect a wide range of hosts in vivo (in the body)..., including human cells in vitro (in test tubes)."

Science 1981;213(4511):1014-1016

resulted in signs of overdose.[87]

Vitamin D overdose has been tied to milk in the United States, which in some cases had 500 times more vitamin D than regulations permit.[83] Other samples didn't have enough vitamin D to even detect any levels.[88]

Because of how large amounts of milk are fortified, vitamin D content of individual samples can vary significantly. Because of these variances and toxicity problems, Britain stopped fortifying milk years ago.[89]

While our vitamin D needs can normally be achieved through exposure to sunlight,

Bovine leukemia virus (BLV) antibodies were present in 59% of newborn calves tested.

Canadian J of Comparative Medicine 1979;43(2):173-179

many commercial cereals like Cheerios, Grapenuts, Raisin Bran, and others are good fortified sources.

The Leukemia/Lymphoma Link

We've talked about milk's possible link to diseases such as osteoporosis, heart disease, and various cancers, but other serious diseases may also be linked to milk consumption. One of those diseases is a major cancer-killer of children, leukemia.

Epidemiological and cluster studies worldwide show leukemia to be more common in the higher dairy consuming populations[90] and where dairy herds are present.[91]

In 1968, a 16-year-old son of a dairy farmer died of lymphosarcoma progressing to acute lymphocytic leukemia.[92]

Ten years earlier, an employee of the same farmer died of lymphosarcoma that progressed to chronic lymphocytic leukemia.[92]

A case of chronic lymphocytic leukemia was also found in a neighbor whose property bordered that farmer's land. Upon investigation, it was discovered that the neighbor had leased some of his own land to the farmer for grazing his herd.[92]

Shortly after the investigation began, a second neighbor was diagnosed with chronic lymphocytic leukemia. The dairy herd, consisting of 250 Holstein cows, had a history of lymphosarcoma occuring at the rate of about one or two cows per year for many years.[92]

Human T-cell leukemia virus can be transmitted from humans to animals. Such results suggest that a milk-borne infection being transferred from a mother to her baby is very plausible. Whether it can pass from a cow to a human is being studied.

Japanese Journal of Cancer Research 1985;76(6):481-487

Community Cancer

Between 1970 and 1973, seven cases of acute lymphocytic leukemia were diagnosed in Elmwood, Wisconsin, representing a 20-fold increase in expected incidence.[93] A number of those who contracted the disease either worked at or lived near the town creamery.

The researchers in this study noted that morphologic similarities existed in the blast cells from all the patients. They wrote: "This cluster of cases may bear a relationship to bovine leukemia since the town was located in dairy farming country and because a number of the patients had either worked at or lived near the town creamery."[93]

Milk powder and whey from the creamery occasionally pervaded the air and even frosted the trees.[93]

Another study of Wisconsin residents re-

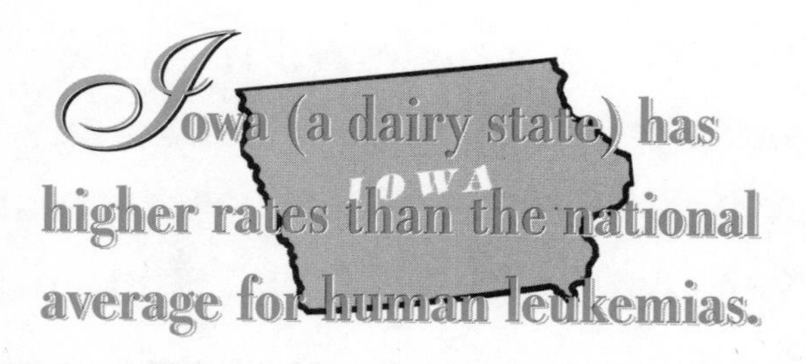

American Journal of Epidemiology 1980;112(1):80-92

Pennsylvania veterinarians have been able to grow BLV in human cells in the laboratory. A 1980 study showed an increase in human leukemia in areas with high levels of bovine leukemia.

Science 1981;213(4511):1014-1016.

vealed "significantly elevated risks (for developing leukemia) among farmers from counties with heavy dairy production."[94]

ALL: The Facts

A study looking at Iowa residents found "a high positive correlation"[95] between males with acute lymphoid leukemia (ALL) and cattle density.[95]

The researchers wrote: "This relationship is greater for dairy cattle than for beef cattle. There is an additional positive relationship between counties with excessive ALL and the presence of dairy herds affected with bovine lymphosarcoma."[95]

In fact, according to the study, 66% of the

Cows infected with BLV had "significantly greater milk production" than their non-BLV infected herdmates,[A] which could mean that more BLV-tainted milk is being produced than previously estimated.

Proceedings of the National Academy of Science of USA 1989;86(3):993-996

ALL cases were seen in those counties with large numbers of dairy cattle and reported bovine leukemia virus (BLV).[95]

In Connecticut, eight members of a farm family who had frequent contact with a BLV-infected herd were diagnosed with cancer.[96]

Pasteur-al Care?

Because of such findings, some researchers are now conducting investigtations to see if bovine leukemia virus is capable of infecting humans through pasteurized milk.[97] While no conclusive evidence has been reported, the BLV virus has been found in meat and unpasteurized milk.[98]

The incidence of BLV varies from herd to

herd, but dairy herds having 80% or more infected adult animals is not uncommon.[99]

In Germany, one researcher tested a herd of 286 Holstein-Freisen cattle every two weeks for four years to track the spread of BLV infection. In the study period, the incidence of infection rose from 4.8% of the herd to 52.6%.[97]

In Florida, 48% of 7,768 dairy cattle were found to have antibodies to BLV.[100] This represented the second-highest BLV concentration rate in the world, next to Venezuela.[100]

In California, now the United States' largest dairy-producing state[101], the number of ma-

Studies linking milk drinking to various cancers are strengthened by evidence that working in close proximity to diseased livestock may increase cancer risk. The study below is one example.

When compared to the general population, veterinarians had a "significantly high" death rate from leukemia and Hodgkin's disease, and from cancers of the brain and skin.

International Journal of Cancer 1980;25(2):181-85

ture cows slaughtered in 1990 for bovine lymphosarcoma caused by BLV was triple the number in 1975.[102]

Because of their own BLV eradication programs and the potential for recontamination, the European Community and other nations will not import U.S. cattle or embryos infected with the virus.[103] Unfortunately, the United States has no BLV eradication program at this time.

Retro Invaders

Bovine leukemia virus is classified as a retrovirus. Retroviruses are unique because they can recode, or reprogram, normal cells to produce more of the invading virus. For human T-cell leukemia virus, a retrovirus,

"Quote"

The present data indicate that MS patients exhibit an... antibody activity against BLV.

Acta Neurologica Scandinavica 1990;81(3):223-228

Many amyotrophic lateral sclerosis (Lou Gerhig disease) patients reported consuming "large quantities of milk."

Neurology 1976;26(2):167-172

mother's milk is "the major route of infection."[104]

The same is true for dairy cows who harbor the bovine form of the disease. Can cow's milk pass such diseases on to humans? At least one journal is stating that animal retroviruses can, indeed, "infect human infants, either as whole virions (viruses) or through reassortment with human or other animal group A rotavi-ruses"[105] thus putting them at risk.

Milk & MS

Now, several studies have reported that a link may exist between milk consumption and multiple sclerosis (MS).[106] One group of researchers concluded that the possible relationship between cow's milk consumption and MS was "highly significant."[107] "A low but still sig-

(Continued on p. 74)

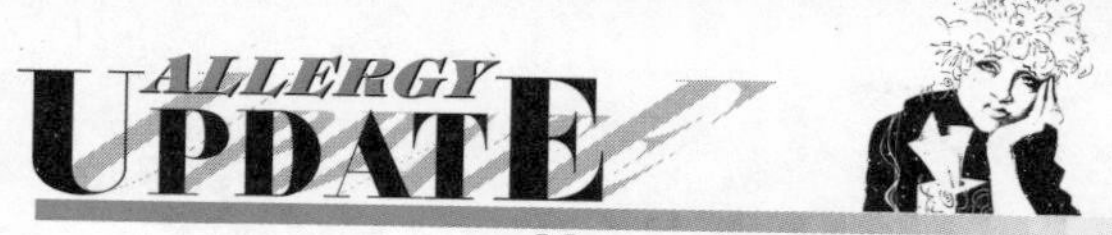

More on the dairy/allergy connection

The information below is but a small sampling of the more than 700 articles published since 1980 on the milk/allergy connection.

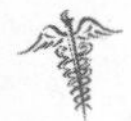

"The symptoms of milk allergy are frequently delayed in appearing, thereby obscuring their connection with the previously ingested food."

- Journal of Family Practice 1979;9(2):223-232

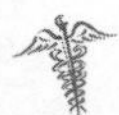

"Allergy to cow's milk may cause disturbances and feeding difficulties. The symptoms include diarrhea, intestinal bleeding, and occult blood in the stools."

- J of Pediatric Gastroenterology and Nutrition 1993;17:451-452

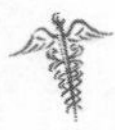

Symptoms of milk-protein allergy include eczema, pylorospasm (stomach problem), colic, cough, choking, gasping, nose colds, constipation, asthma, anorexia, sneezing attacks, vomiting, headaches, and fatigue.

- Annals of Allergy 1951;9:195
- Lancet 1978;1(8059):304-305

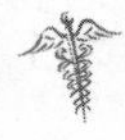

"Milk allergy is not confined to infancy, but is frequently seen in children and adults, often persisting as an allergy which had supposedly been 'outgrown.'"

- Journal of Family Practice 1979;9(2):223-232

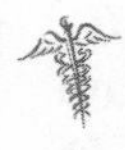

Researchers in Poland studied 153 infants with pneumonia and/or bronchitis suspected to be allergic to cow's milk. 62.7% of the children were confirmed to be allergic, which represented "20.8% of hospitalized infants" with respiratory tract diseases.

- Roczniki Akademii Medycznej W Bialymstoku 1995;40(3):433-8

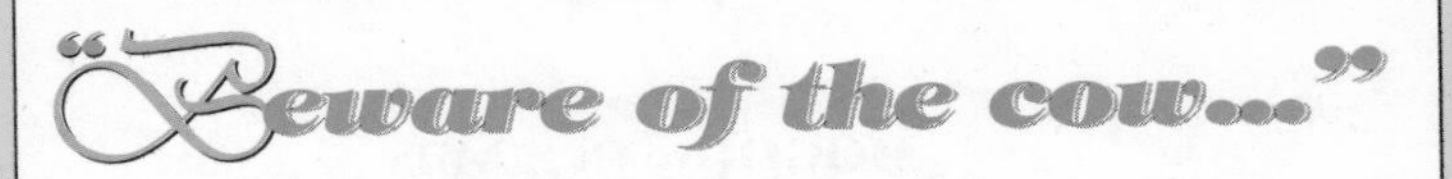

So warned an editorial in The Lancet. A valid warning? Before deciding, consider milk's possible link with:

- **Multiple sclerosis** *(Lancet 1974;2:1061; Neuroepidemiology 1992;11:304-312)*
- **Leukemia** *(Science 1981;213:1014)*
- **Lou Gehrig's Disease** *(Neurology 1976;26(2):167-72)*
- **Nephrosis (kidney disease)** *(Clinical Research 1975;74A)*
- **Pediatric "growing pains"** *(Don't Drink Your Milk, page 31)*
- **Streptococcal infections** *(Ibid, page 32)*
- **Allergy-induced bedwetting** *(Pediatr Clin North Amer 1975;22:227-38)*
- **Pediatric hyperactivity** *(Don't Drink Your Milk, page 87)*
- **Learning difficulties** *(Pediatr Clin North Amer 1975;22:227-38)*
- **Tension Fatigue Syndrome** *(Pediatr Clin North Amer 1975;22:227-38)*
- **Chronic diarrhea & GI upset** *(Pediatrics 1967;40:354)*
- **Vomiting, eczema, bronchitis** *(Acta Paediatr Scand (Supp) 1973;234.)*
- **Juvenile Atherosclerosis** *(Curr Probl Pediatr 1979;9(3):1-38)*
- **Ischemic Heart Disease** *(Int'l Journal of Cardiology 1994;46:197-207)*
- **Female Infertility** *(American Journal of Epidemiology 1994;139(3):282-9)*
- **Ulcerative colitis** *(Israel J of Medical Sciences 1985;21:575)*
- **Lupus erythematosus** *(Rheumatic Disease Clinics of North Amer 1988;14(1):15)*
- **Cataracts** *(Digestive Diseases and Sciences 1982;27(3):257-64)*
- **Infant colic** *(Pediatrics 1991;87:439)*
- **Stomach pain and cramping** *(Medical Tribune 1993;34:21)*

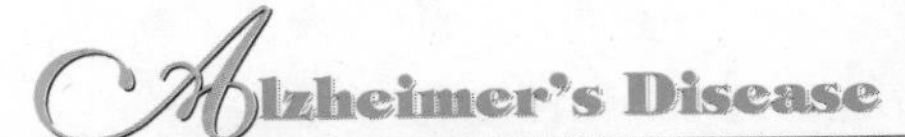

"Some of the 4 million people in the United States suffering from Alzheimer's may actually be infected with the agent that causes CJD (Creutzfeldt-Jakob Disease). And that raises the question: Has an unrecognized form of BSE (bovine spongiform encephalopathy) infected US cattle and entered the human food chain?"

Neurologia 1995;10(1):37-40;10(4):177; 1995;10(5):213-214

nificant correlation" was found for cream and butter consumption and MS.[107]

In one study, researchers found "significant correlations between 1. cow milk production per inhabitant, 2. national bovine density per inhabitant, and 3. local bovine geographic density, and MS prevalence."[108]

Scientists already know that polio virus, myxovirus, hepatitis virus, foot and mouth disease virus, and tick-borne encephalitis are all milk-transmissible diseases. Foot and mouth disease virus, Maloney leukemia virus, Rauscher's leukemia virus and Rous sarcoma virus can all survive pasteurization.[109]

The bovine leukemia virus is a tumor-inducing virus that can affect other animals.[110]

By Federal law, 1 cc (about 1/5 tsp) of grade A pasteurized milk can contain 750,000 lymphocytes and other blood cells—and still be sold.

Environmental Nutrition 1994 January

Lymphoma was histopathologically diagnosed in 86% of cows from one herd that tested positive for BLV antibodies.

J of the National Cancer Institute 1985;74(3):711-714

Newborn sheep inoculated with BLV became infected with the disease, and 50% of them died with histologically confirmed tumors.[110]

When experimental animals that have died of BLV are autopsied, cancer cells have been found in the bone marrow, spleen, lymph nodes, lungs, liver, heart, stomach, spinal cord, kidneys, and behind the eyes.[111,112]

BLV has been transmitted both orally and by injection of infected lymphoctyes to chickens, sheep, goats, rabbits, pigs, rats, Rhesus monkeys, chimpanzees, and other mammals.[113]

It's sobering to consider that according to Federal law, US Grade A milk can contain up to 750,000 lymphocytes, or pus cells, and other types of blood cells, and still be sold for human consumption.

BLV In You & Me?

Can BLV be passed to humans, too? No one knows yet, but investigators are looking at the issue more closely.

In the past, there was no evidence that BLV

could infect humans. But since the advent of more sophisticated genetic testing called polymerase chain reaction testing, BLV antibodies have been found in humans. Such antibodies suggest the possibility of BLV cross-infections.[114]

Viral pathogens, or virus germs, are capable of being transmitted by both human and animal nursing mothers. Most BLV-infected cows release infectious viruses and infected lymphocytes (white blood cells) in their milk.[115]

Many cows that are removed from herds because of poor performance (they don't give enough milk), or for other reasons, have been found to have leukemia, or at least show evidence of the disease.[116]

"It is concluded that milk transmission of BLV (from cow to calf) is responsible in part for the high rates of infection encountered in our dairy herds..."

Tropical Animal Health and Production 1983;15(4):215-218

"QUOTE"

These data confirm the presence of BIV in milk and identify the potential for lactogenic (milk) transmission of the virus.

American Journal of Veterinary Research 1995;56(4):445-449

BIV = HIV?

Milk-borne transmission of the AIDS retrovirus has been documented in both humans and dairy cows.[104,117] The bovine immunodeficiency virus (BIV) has been detected in blood tests in beef and dairy cattle in the United States, Europe, Australia, and New Zealand.[117] In one test with cattle from the Mississippi Agriculture and Forestry Experiment Station, infection rates were higher than 50%.[118]

This could be very serious since the cow AIDS virus is very similar to the human AIDS virus. Can it be transferred from cow to consumer? We don't know for sure yet. The USDA has, however, transferred BIV infection from cattle to goats, sheep, and rabbits by blood transfer.[119]

We do know that BLV has been transferred to chimpanzees through milk.[120] The chimpanzees drank milk known to be infected with BLV and both died with confirmed erythroleukemia and Pneumocystis carinii pneumonia—a hallmark of AIDS infections.[120]

The first case of a confirmed BIV infection in humans was reported in 1992.[121]

Bovine leukemia virus and bovine immunodeficiency virus are related to the only known human retroviruses: human T-cell leukemia virus, and HIV, or human AIDS.[119]

Government researchers say that BIV and

Environmental Nutrition, January, 1994

Just because raw milk is "certified," it is no guarantee that it is germ-free.

RAW

MILK

1 LITER

"QUOTE"

Milk and milk products have been implicated in the transmission of human pathogens, including salmonella.

Journal of Dairy Science 1992;75:2327

BLV pose no threat to human health. Others, including Dr. Virgil Hulse, a research physician, epidemiologist, former dairy inspector, and specialist in the area of milk and dairy, believe that further studies are needed.

SAY CHEESE?

Bacterial and viral contamination pose a real problem for milk and dairy product consumers. Only 38% of the milk used to make cheese is subjected to any heat treatment.[122] In the United States, cheeses made from underpasteurized or unpasteurized milk require an aging process to prevent the survival of pathogenic bacteria.[123] How successful this aging process is has not been sufficiently tested to guarantee its safety and effectiveness.

Emmenthal, Camembert, Roquefort, Gruyere, and some other cheeses are difficult,

> ***"Salmonella are widespread in the environment and hence can enter the dairy factory from various sources."***
>
> *Journal of Dairy Science 1992;75:2338*

if not impossible, to make from milk heated to or above pasteurization temperature.[124] Because of this, milk used for most cheese manufacturing is heated to temperatures below what is required for pasteurization.[124]

While pasteurization is important for making cottage cheese and other soft cheeses, they may be contaminated *after* pasteurization, and high coliform bacteria counts are often found in them.[125]

Salmonella-Slices?

In 1989, Mozzarella cheese and shredded cheese products were identified by epidemiological evidence as the vehicles of infection in an outbreak of salmonellosis in Minnesota and Wisconsin.[126]

In 1980, more than 339 cases of salmonella poisoning traced to cheddar cheese were reported in Colorado.[127]

A massive outbreak of salmonellosis involving more than 180,000 people in the midwestern U.S. in 1985 was traced to 2% fat, pasteurized fluid milk that allegedly became contaminated *after* pasteurization.[128]

Two outbreaks of salmonellosis in Canada, one in 1982 and the other in 1984, were both tied to contaminated cheese.[129]

A nationwide outbreak of salmonellosis occurred in the U.S. in September of 1994, and

The RAW Facts

Meaningful differences in nutritional value between pasteurized and unpasteurized (raw) milk have not been demonstrated, and other purported benefits of raw milk have not been substantiated. Conversely, the role of unpasteurized dairy products in the transmission of infectious diseases has been established repeatedly.

Journal of the American Medical Association 1984;252(15):2048-52 was traced to contaminated ice cream.[130] The ice cream premix had been pasteurized, but was transported in trailers that had just carried nonpasteurized liquid eggs.[130] The outbreak affected 224,000 people[130], with symptoms varying from mild to very severe.

These are just a few of the many cases that could be cited. In commenting on several outbreaks of salmonella traced to milk or cheese, one researcher wrote that "use of contaminated raw materials or ingredients, improper or insufficient processing, and post-processing contamination were among the probable causes."[131]

Another researcher wrote: "Cheese and other similar food items may be more common sources of apparently sporadic salmonella infections than previously recognized."[132]

Researchers have reported that salmonella

Many diseases such as tuberculosis, brucellosis, diphtheria, scarlet fever, Q-fever, and gastroenteritis are transmissible by milk products.

Journal of Dairy Science 1988;71:2809-2816

Milk is an excellent vehicle of infection because its fat content protects pathogens from gastric acid, and, being fluid, it has a relatively short gastric transit time.

Journal of the American Medical Association 1984;252:2048-52

survived in ripening Cheddar cheese for 7 months at 53°F and for 10 months at 44°F.[132]

1 + 1 = 58?

Polio virus and other viruses have been found to survive the aging process used in producing cottage cheese curd, cheddar cheese, and sour milk products.[133] While pasteurization is protective, some researchers feel that the nucleic acid, or genetic material of the viral agent, could possibly recombine with healthy host cells to produce more of the invading virus![134]

Such viruses are not the only potential problem. "Despite ultra high temperature, milk and milk products might still contain bacterial fragments which could produce an allergenic or activating role on the immune system."[135] The government estimates that foodborne diseases affect as many as 33 million people a year, killing up to 9,000.[136]

Each year, more than 40,000 Salmonella infections are reported to the Center for Disease Control in Atlanta.[137] This number, however, represents just a fraction of the actual infections in the US,[138] representing "only the tip of the iceberg" of the salmonella epidemic.[139]

Some estimates put the total number of salmonella cases each year in the US at 2 million![140]

Transmission Troubles

But this concern is nothing new. Disease-causing bacteria in milk have been a matter of public health concern since the early days of dairy production. Tuberculosis, brucellosis, diphtheria, scarlet fever, Q-fever, and gastroenteritis are all transmissible by milk products.[141]

Septic arthritis, caused by Streptococcus lactis, has been positively associated with the use of unpasteurized milk.[142] Pasteurization

(Continued on p. 86)

The Cream of the Crop?

Is our milk supply the best it can possibly be? Well,... Consumer's Union sampled milk from processing plants in Iowa, Illinois, Kansas, Arkansas, and Missouri. Their report was rather sour, concluding that "the milk supply throughout the area covered in our test poses a potential hazard." What did they find?

Taste

Investigators tasted at least 3 samples from each of 25 brands and found that:

- Only 12% of samples were free from taste-compromising defects
- Different samples from the same brand had widely different tastes*
- One third contained flavors of feed recently fed to the cows
- Many samples tasted "cooked," a result of sloppy processing
- Many tasted "flat" (may have absorbed container chemicals)

*Would you be concerned if your tap water tasted different regularly?

Additives

What "extras" did investigators find?

- Only four of 25 samples had no detectable pesticide level
- 21 samples contained residues of chlorinated hydrocarbons

Bacteria

Government regulations permit pasteurized milk to have up to 750,000 lymphocytes, 20,000 bacteria, and 10 coliform organisms per 1/5 teaspoon—about 8 drops! But at 40° F, the temperature of a good refrigerator, the population of those "bugs" can double every 35-40 hours! Investigators found seven milk samples with more than 130,000 bacteria per 1/5 teaspoon, and one sample had "too many to count." How many does your milk have?

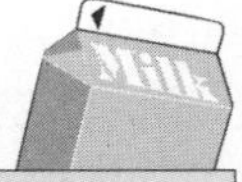

In Their Own Words...

> "The quality of a number of the dairy products in this study was little short of deplorable."

Consumer Reports, January, 1974, "Why is the Quality of Milk So Low?"

Listeria organisms excreted in cow's milk escaped pasteurization, grew well at refrigerator temperatures, and were ingested (by consumers).

"QUOTE"

New England Journal of Medicine 1985;312(7):439

helps, but numerous recalls of milk, cheese, and ice cream have aroused new concerns over the safety of our milk supply.[141]

Pasteurization Problems?

In 1983, pasteurized whole milk was implicated as a source of a listeriosis outbreak that occurred in Massachusetts.[143] The authors of a report about that incident stated: "These results support the hypothesis that human listeriosis can be a food-borne disease and raise questions about the ability of pasteurization to eradicate a large inoculum of (listeriosis) from contaminated raw milk."[143]

The authors also stated that the milk "implicated in this outbreak was apparently properly pasteurized"[143] and couldn't say when it became contaminated.

In 1985, 142 cases of listeriosis resulting in 48 deaths in Los Angeles County, California, were traced to Mexican-style cheese contaminated with L. monocytogenes from unpasteurized milk.[144] Twenty fetuses, 10 neonates, and 18 adults died from the disease.[144]

Adding further concern to this issue, a commentary on this report stated: "The excretion of Listeriosis monocytogenes in cow's milk is well recognized. Cows with listeric mastitis may produce normal-appearing milk containing large numbers of bacteria. Some of the organisms may survive pasteurization and then grow better (faster) than competing species at refrigerator temperatures—a phenomenon called 'cold enrichment.' Milk may be a

QUOTE

These results support the hypothesis that human listeriosis can be a foodborne disease and raise questions about the ability of pasteurization to eradicate a large inoculum of listeria from contaminated raw milk.

New England Journal of Medicine 1985;312(7):404

particularly effective vehicle because it protects the bacteria from gastric acid."[145]

Listeriosis can cause meningitis, endocarditis (inflammation of heart membrane), stillbirths, spontaneous abortion, and inflammatory lesions.

Listeria bacteria are found in human and animal excrement and in animal silage. Exposure to listeria produces similar diseases in both humans and animals.

While improper pasteurization can be a cause, other reports suggest that listeria is relatively resistant to heat treatments.[146] Such evidence calls into question the effectiveness of even the best pasteurization methods.

A number of outbreaks of Yersinia enterocolitica, another bacterial contaminant,

Vaccinations against Q-fever in a herd of goats in France did not prevent the disease, which was passed from their milk to consumers.

Am Journal of Tropical Medicine and Hygiene 1992;47(1):35-40

"QUOTE"

Butter readily supports growth of salmonella at room temperature, but refrigeration or freezing for brief periods does not eliminate it. Salmonella can remain viable in butter for up to 9 months.

Journal of Dairy Science 1992;75(9):2339

have been tied to the consumption of pasteurized chocolate milk and regular milk.[147] Symptoms include arthritis, acute gastroenteritis (inflammation of the GI tract), septicemia (blood poisoning), and swollen lymph nodes.[148]

Should We Call it No-Gurt?

Salmonella and E coli contamination of animal products continues to be a serious problem for the food industry. Since proper pasteurization kills these pathogens, most salmonella and E coli contamination of dairy products has been associated with raw milk, cheese, raw eggs, or yogurt containing live cultures.[149]

In fact, at a recent meeting of the American College of Gastroenterology, investigators presented well-documented case reports of serious gastrointestinal diseases caused by eating live yogurt bacteria.[150]

"It is reasonable to conjecture that M. paratuberculosis may be responsible for some cases of Crohn's disease."

Journal of Clinical Microbiology 1992;30(12):3070-3073

One man developed autoimmune chronic active hepatitis after eating 16 ounces of yogurt with live cultures daily for one year.[150] Yogurt can also worsen the condition of patients with inflammatory bowel disease.[150]

In spite of precautions, numerous outbreaks of infection have been associated with pasteurized products.[149] Milk casein tends to promote bacterial growth, making proper pasteurization, handling, and refrigeration of milk a critical public health issue.

The Crohn's Connection

Now, a possible link between Johne's disease in cattle and Crohn's disease in humans is being studied. Mycobacterium paratuberculosis (M. paratuberculosis) is the highly contagious, infectious agent responsible for Johne's disease, which is characterized by severe bowel inflammation, diarrhea, malnutrition, and eventual death.[151]

Current medical practice is to treat Crohn's disease with anti-inflammatory drugs. Such a practice is consistent with the prevailing opinion that a major component, if not the cause of the disease, is autoimmune related.[152]

Autoimmunity is a condition characterized by an immune response of the body against its own tissues—like the apparent ability of milk protein to stimulate the body to attack the insulin-producing cells of the pancreas which can cause the onset of juvenile diabetes.

There are between 20,000 and 25,000 new Crohn's cases reported each year[152], and that

"Johne's disease and Crohn's disease are remarkably similar in clinical signs and intestinal pathology."

Hoard's Dairyman, January 25, 1995, p. 43

number is rising. It normally affects people who are 15 to 30 years old, and may come from exposure "to an agent or environmental factor or factors in early childhood."[152]

Crohn's disease, which mimics Johne's disease, has long been suspected of having a link with the animal form of the disease.[153]

Research has shown that M. paratuberculosis is found in the milk of cows infected with Johne's disease.[154] M. paratuberculosis can withstand exposure to very high temperatures and thus can survive pasteurization far better than other mycobacteria.[155]

The Chain Reaction

Through polymerase chain reaction testing, human tissue samples from Crohn's patients have revealed the presence of DNA sequences specific to M. paratuberculosis.[156]

Two-thirds of the intestine samples from 40 Crohn's patients revealed evidence of the mycobacterium, but less than 5% of intestinal samples from 23 ulcerative colitis patients contained it.[157]

A random sample of 54 Wisconsin dairy herds found 50% of the herds testing positive for the M. paratuberculosis bacterium.[158]

Dr. Mike Collins, a research veterinarian at the University of Wisconsin School of Veterinary Medicine, specializes in Johne's disease. He says that "recent information suggests that Mycobacterium paratuberculosis is more widely spread than previously thought, and could be a food-borne pathogen, confounding occupational risk factors."[152]

In Collins' laboratory, pasteurization time required to kill 100% of one strain of M. paratuberculosis was 9 minutes.[152] Normal industry pasteurization time is 15 seconds.[152,159]

Some factors linking Crohn's disease and M. paratuberculosis are:[152]

"QUOTE"

Of 77 milk samples (taken from cows with Johne's disease), 11.6% were culture-positive (contained M. paratuberculosis).

Journal of Clinical Microbiology 1992;30(1):166-171

1. Isolation of M. paratuberculosis from a patient with Crohn's disease was reported in 1984. The isolate, when orally inoculated into infant goats, caused Johne's disease;

2. Since 1984, isolation of M. paratuberculosis from Crohn's patients has been reported from almost every developed country in the world;

3. In 1992, using newly developed genetic probes, researchers reported that 65% of Crohn's patients studied had M. paratuberculosis in their intestinal tissues.

Such evidence is significant, but more studies are needed to establish a link between Johne's disease and Crohn's disease.

M. paratuberculosis-specific DNA strains were isolated in 13 of 18 samples of children with Crohn's disease.

Journal of Infectious Disease 1994;169(2):449-451

"QUOTE"

The evidence for a relationship between Johne's disease and Crohn's disease...is sufficiently strong enough that all dairy farmers should be aware of what is known—and unknown.

Johne's disease expert Dr. Michael Collins, quoted in *Hoard's Dairyman*, January 25, 1995, p. 43

Bovine Barnyard Blunders

Here's another troubling trend from the bovine barnyard. It has been estimated that one-half of the 30 million pounds of antibiotics produced annually in the United States is given to animals. Many of those animals are eaten by humans, who may be taking antibiotics themselves—often unnecessarily.

Some researchers say that between 50-60% of prescription drugs for outpatients are inappropriate.[160] According to Dr. Alexander Tomasz, of Rockefeller University in New York and a leading authority on antibiotic-resistant

In 1992, 19,000 deaths were attributed to infections caused by antiobiotic-resistant orgranisms. They played a partial role in another 58,000 deaths that same year.

Your Health, June, 1994

bacteria, this antibiotic abuse is threatening a chilling, post-antibiotic era that would be "nothing short of a medical disaster."[161]

Super Drugs=Super Bugs?

Dr. Tomasz says that only the most antibiotic-resistant strains of "bugs" are surviving.[161] Doctors are concerned about drug-resistant strains of pneumococcus, tuberculosis, staphylococcus, and enterococcal pathogens causing untreatable infections. If you get one of these strains, Dr. Tomasz says, "you are in the hands of the Almighty."[161]

A Government Accounting Office report indicated that the FDA tests for just four of the 82 drugs that are commonly used in milk cows.[162] According to the GAO, 35 of the most commonly used drugs for cows have never been approved for use in dairy cows.[162] The report also said that those drugs are being used routinely, not just in emergencies.

While the law prohibits using animal drugs in any manner aside from those specified on the label, the FDA created a loophole in 1984 to let doctors in emergencies treat animals with

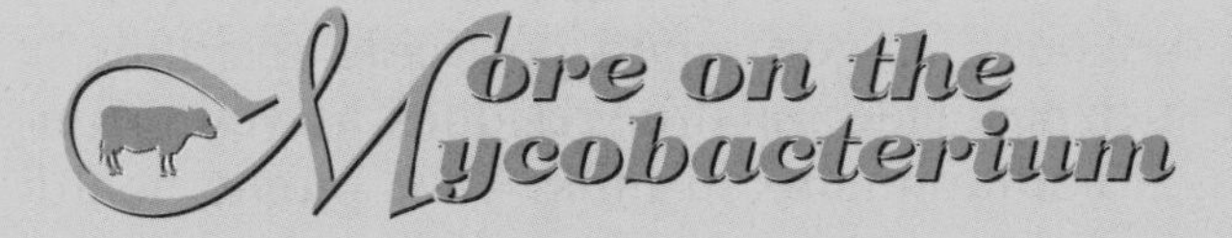

Johne's disease expert Dr. Michael Collins made the following statements during the 1994 meeting of the United States Animal Health Association.

"While the evidence for a causal relationship between M. paratuberculosis and Crohn's disease is not yet overwhelming, it is sufficiently strong that animal industries and the United States Animal Health Association should take action."

"If M. paratuberculosis becomes established as the cause of Crohn's disease, or even an important complicating infectious agent,...(its) magnitude as a food safety issue will be profound."

"M. paratuberculosis is known to be excreted in the milk of infected cows."

drugs not labeled for their use. Thus, in an emergency, drugs approved for use in horses could be used for cows.[162]

MILK'S ADDED "EXTRAS"

A 1988 FDA survey of milk samples from grocery stores in 10 cities found that 73% of the samples contained pesticide residues.[163] Such pesticide and drug residues, as well as fungal contaminants in milk, have public health officials concerned, and researchers looking for possible adverse consequences.[163]

Since 1988, three surveys have found illegal residues of sulfamethazine in retail milk supplies in more than a dozen US cities.[163]

Sulfamethazine is a sulfa-based over-the-counter antibiotic widely used in treating ani-

Researchers found residues of sulfamethazine in about 20% of the milk purchased in several major Eastern cities.

The Atlanta Journal/Constitution January 9, 1990

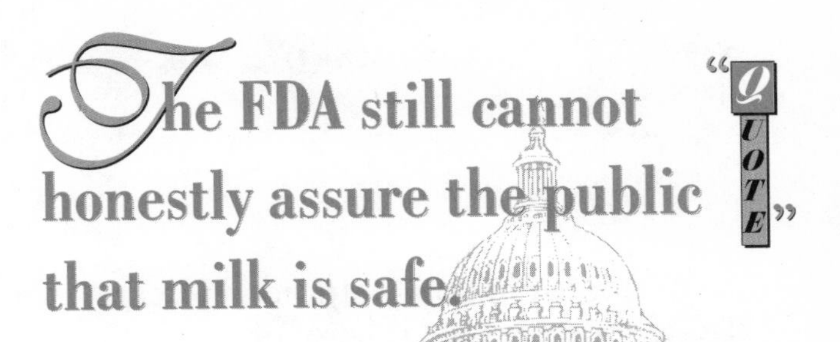

Rep. Ted Weiss, chairman of the House Government Operations Subcommittee on Human Resources. Reported by AP 8/6/1992

mal diseases, but not approved for human use. It is used legally to control bacterial diseases in swine, beef cows, sheep, chickens, and turkeys. There are times, however, when it is used illegally for the same purpose in dairy cows.[163]

Laboratory studies show the drug causes cancer in animals and may affect individuals sensitive to sulfa drugs.[163] Drinking milk contaminated with such drugs could cause children to develop sensitivities to sulfa drugs and not even know it.[163]

This is a very serious problem which is underscored by the fact that FDA scientists say the accidental or deliberate misuse of the drug in a single cow can contaminate the pooled milk of as many as 70,000 cows![163]

Now, the use of synthetic hormones, such as rBGH (recombinant bovine growth hormone) has come under fire because of the increased mastitis (inflamed mammary glands) rates it causes in cows, which then requires even more antibiotic use.[164]

In addition, some studies indicate that rBGH promotes the release of a substance in cow's milk called IGF-1 (insulin-like growth factor). Milk taken from rBGH-treated cows can have IGF-1 levels that are up to 300% higher than milk from a non-rBGH-treated cow.[164]

IGF-1 has not been sufficiently tested to ensure safety in humans, yet the FDA approved it for human ingestion anyway. New evidence, however, is casting serious doubt on its safety, linking even small amounts of IGF-1 to accelerated growth of cancer cells.[164]

According to the research, normally slow cancers that take many decades to grow enough to be detected, could start appearing in just 10-20 years, or even less.[164,165]

(Continued on p. 102.)

The USDA projects that 60% of dairy cows will be receiving rBGH by the year 2000.

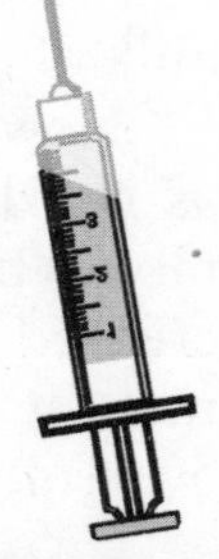

***Consumer Reports*, May 1992, p. 331**

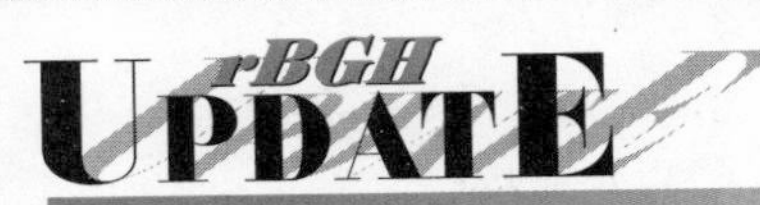

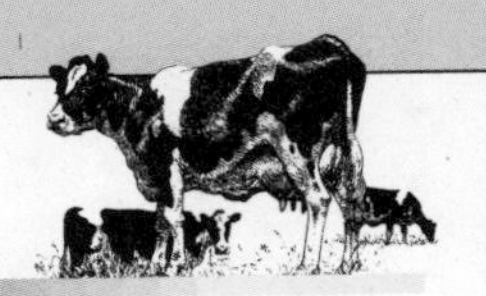

More on the rBGH/IGF-1 controversy

There's a milk glut in the US today, and the government spends hundreds of millions of tax dollars each year to buy the surplus. As a result, many are wondering why rBGH is needed. Others are sounding an alarm about its potential dangers.

In a letter to FDA Commissioner David Kessler, Dr. Samuel Epstein, a professor at the University of Chicago's School of Public Health, expressed his concern about the link between drinking milk from rBGH-treated cows and human breast cancer. Giving cows rBGH, he said, increases their levels of IGF-1, which can cause normal breast epithelial cells to become malignant cancer cells. IGF-1, he said, also encourages breast cancer cell growth.

• Food Safety Week 1994 Feb;56:21-22

Posilac (tradename for rBGH) increases risk of bovine mastitis (udder infection) and "has been associated with increases in somatic (pus) cell counts."

• Package insert warning sent with drug by its maker

The IGF-1 found in cows is chemically identical to that found in humans. rBGH can increase IGF-1 levels by as much as 25% to 300% in cows.

• Consumer Reports, May 1992, p. 331

Human experiments show that IGF-1 exerts "a dramatic protective effect" against cancer cell death. When IGF-1 body levels are decreased, "rapid, massive cancer cell death occurs."

• Cancer Research 1995;55:2463-2469

Milk producers are not required to specially label milk telling consumers it contains rBGH. Only four states (Vermont, Minnesota, Wisconsin, Maine) have passed laws making it legal for rBGH-free milk to be specially labeled as such.

According to cancer researcher Dr. George Tritsch, IGF-1 can stimulate normally slow-growing cancers (like breast, ovarian, and prostate) to grow very quickly, causing them to appear "in a decade or two or even less."

Delicious 12/95, p. 9

According to cancer researcher Dr. George Tritsch, "increases in IGF-1 at such low levels could readily enter the bloodstream of individuals drinking milk from rBGH-treated cows."[164]

One recent study reported that the presence of IGF-1 may play "a very important protective role"[165] in preventing cancer cell destruction, while simultaneously promoting tumor growth and aggressiveness.[165] When IGF-1 levels were decreased, "massive (cancer) cell death" occurred.[165]

Another infectious agent, which does not fall into the category of a virus or bacteria, is receiving special attention from many scientists. Known as prions, or proteinaceous infectious particles, they are responsible for the *prion diseases*, or fatal spongiform encephalopathies.[166]

These degenerative diseases riddle the brain with holes, making it look something like Swiss cheese. The resulting gradual dementia and eventual death is unavoidable, because there is no cure.

BSE, TME, and CJD

The most common forms are scrapie disease in sheep, bovine spongiform encephalopathy (BSE, or mad cow disease), transmissible mink encephalopathy (TME), and Creutzfeldt-Jakob disease (CJD) in humans.

In the late 1970s and early 80s, an epidemic of *mad cow disease* raged through England as a result of rendering, or feeding dead, scrapie-

"It may be 10-15 years before it can be determined with any certainty that BSE does represent a risk to the human population."

QUOTE

The New Scientist, June 16, 1990

British scientists have now shown that mad cow disease and Creutzfeldt-Jakob Disease "show very close genetic similarities."

Nature 1996;380(6576):675

infected sheep to cows as a protein supplement.[167] About 100,000 cows have been diagnosed with the disease to date.

Prions: Mysterious Mutators

Dr. Sheila Gore of the Biostatistics Unit of the Medical Research Council in England says that by April of 1995, BSE had been confirmed in 53% of Britain's dairy herds.[168]

"Taken together," Dr. Gore says, "cases of Creutzfeldt-Jakob disease in farmers and young adults are more than happenstance."[168]

According to one report, "some researchers estimate that nearly 34 million beef-eating humans may have been exposed. They say the incubation period could range up to 30 years," which means it could be a long time before cases start turning up in large numbers.[168,169]

In 1988, Britain banned the sale of ruminant (cows', goats', etc.) brains and organs for human consumption.[170] Similar bans have been imposed in Ireland, France, and Switzerland, where the disease has also been found.[170]

Members of a Jewish group in Libya who eat sheep eyes and brains have developed a form of CJD, and some inhabitants of a rural area of Czechoslovakia with known sheep scrapie cases have also contracted CJD.[171]

Defective Neighbors

Scientists argued for quite some time whether prions were capable of infecting other proteins. Then, geneticist Susan Lindquist at

Rendering The Facts...

Dr. David Taylor of Edinburgh University (Britain), took brain matter from scrapie-infected sheep, subjected it to a rendering process, and injected it into the brains of mice. Many of the mice contracted a similar disease. Dr. Taylor says that none of the several rendering processes he tried stopped the scrapie transfer completely. This is proof, he said, that common methods of rendering animals for use in animal feed are ineffective in destroying the agent that causes scrapie.

Reuters News Service, May 13, 1996

the University of Chicago, found that proteins with defective traits similar to the prions thought to cause mad cow disease were, indeed, capable of passing their defects to the proteins in neighboring cells.[172]

"(That prions can indeed affect and mutate surrounding proteins) is a plausible mechanism now," Lindquist said in an interview with Reuters.[173] "If you can see it working in yeast, it makes it plausible that it could work in other proteins."

GENE GENIES?

She said she believes the deformed protein "cozied up" to proteins in other cells, forcing them to adopt the same deformed shape. It was the first time characteristics of proteins

"QUOTE"

There is evidence that the temperatures reached during pasteurization of milk and processing or cooking meat do not inactivate (prions.)

Proceedings of the U.S. Animal Health Association 1988;413-415

Doctors at a VA hospital in Pennsylvania autopsied 54 demented patients and discovered that 5.5% had died of CJD, a rate of occurrence about 1,000 times higher than expected.

Neurology 1989;39(1):76-79

have been shown to pass from one protein to another without DNA undergoing any change. "It's genetics without DNA," Lindquist said.[173]

In another Reuters report, British government scientists said they found evidence that mad cow disease can be passed from cow to calf, but probably not through milk since dairy calves do not normally drink their mother's milk.[174] More investigations are being conducted on this issue.

Reuters also reported that a British coroner ruled that a young 20-year-old vegetarian who died of CJD caught it from eating tainted hamburgers as a child.[175]

Because of such findings, researchers say that "a link between scrapie and Creutzfeldt-Jakob disease is likely to exist."[176]

While most mad cow research to date has

been done with meat eating, it raises the question of whether prion problems could come from milk as well.

Prions: Irresistable?

The possibility of cross-species infection is not surprising since prions do not have DNA or RNA, but multiply by mutating normal proteins into dangerous ones. As a result, the body cannot produce antibodies to resist or destroy prions.

Prions cannot be cultured in a laboratory test, and have survived temperatures of 360° centigrade for 1 hour.[177] These high temperatures for such a length of time would require the rendering industry to use cooking proce-

(Continued on p. 110.)

CJD has apparently been transmitted by cornea transplants, brain electrodes, surgical instruments, and injection of human growth hormone.

Scientific American 1995;272(1):48-51

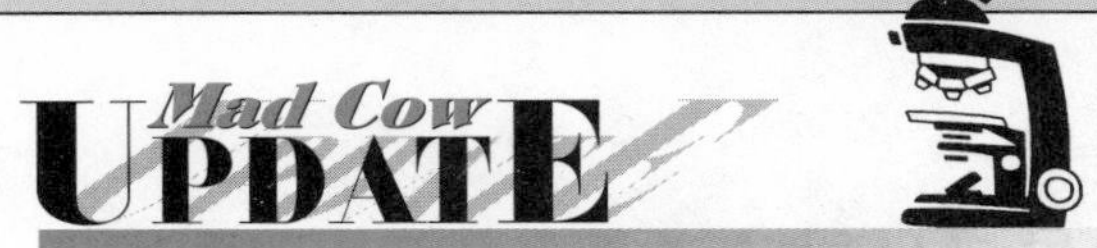

More on the BSE/CJD controversy

The government says there's no BSE danger in the U.S. But according to Robert Rohwer, director of molecular virology at the VA Medical Center in Baltimore, MD: "The only thing that stands between us and an epidemic is unmitigated luck." (Time 1/27/97, p. 53.) Why are some experts so concerned about the BSE/CJD question?

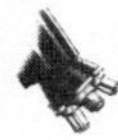

"New variant" Creutzfeldt-Jakob disease has strain characteristics distinct from other types of CJD and which resemble those of BSE transmitted to mice, domestic cat and macaque, consistent with BSE being the source of this new disease.

- Nature 1996;383(6602):685-690

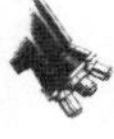

Responding to claims of the safety of British beef in the wake of the BSE outbreak in that country, the United Kingdom medical chief suggested that "safe" does not necessarily mean "no risk."

- Nature 1996;383(6599):371

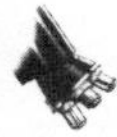

Nonhuman primates inoculated with brain tissue from two humans with Alzheimer's disease developed a spongiform encephalopathy that was "indistinguishable from CJD."

- Neurology 1980;30(9):945-950

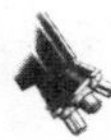

Scrapie-associated fibrils were found in fresh and frozen brains infected with CJD.

- Research in Virology 1992;143(6):387-395

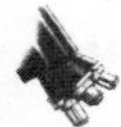

Two British farmers who had "mad cows" in their herds died in 1995 of CJD.

- Scientific American 1995;272(1):48-57

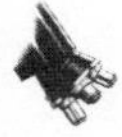

When sheep are inoculated with cells from a CJD-infected human brain, they develop scrapie.

- In These Times 5/31/93, p. 14

> *Ample justification exists for considering a similar pathogensis for Alzheimer's disease and the spongiform virus encephalopathies.*
>
> "QUOTE"
>
> Annals of the New York Academy of Sciences 1982;396:131-143

dures and equipment that are not presently available or practical.[178]

Compounding the problem is the fact that prions are also highly resistant to irradiation.[177]

A Bum Steer?

The USDA has officially declared that no prion disease exists in American cattle. But in Stetsonville, Wisconsin, minks that ate rendered products taken from an infected cow (called a *downer cow* because the disease riddles its brain with holes to the point that the cow can no longer stand up) contracted TME (transmissible mink encephalopathy, the mink form of the disease) in just 7 months.[179]

Of 7,300 minks that ate the rendered products, 60% developed clinical signs of spongiform disease, and all of these eventually died from it.[179]

One farmer who drank milk from his own herd died from Creutzfeldt-Jakob disease.[170]

Investigation revealed that some of his cows were infected with BSE.[170]

In 1989, the United States produced 5.5 million metric tons, or 12.5 billion pounds, of rendered products—dead animals and dead animal parts that have been processed and added to animal feed.[180]

In the United States, renderers pick up 100 million pounds of waste material every day![181] They retrieve a mixture of slaughterhouse and restaurant scraps, and dead farm animals. According to one report, it's a "witches' brew of feet, heads, stomachs, intestines, hooves, spinal cords, tails, grease, feathers, and bones."[181]

Surprisingly, about half of every butchered

Renderers pick up the carcasses of 100,000 downer cows each year for processing into feed supplements and other uses.

N.Y. Times News Service, 3/11/97

cow and a third of every pig is not consumed by humans![181] Much, if not all, of the remains are sold to renderers for disposal.

Udderly Disgusting!

Like it or not, even road kills—possums, squirrels, cats, dogs, and other animals killed by cars and trucks—and euthanized cats and dogs are rendered.[181] The city of Los Angeles alone sends 200 tons of euthanized cats and dogs to West Coast Rendering every month, according to Chuck Ellis, a spokesman for the city's Sanitation Department.[181]

The byproducts of rendering are used for making lubricants, lipstick, cement, polish, inks, waxes, soaps, candles, pharmaceuticals, garden fertilizers, gummy candies, and for enriching animal feeds, including dog and cat food.[181]

Because of widespread use of rendering and because of its consequences in Britain and Europe, it is imperative that further studies be conducted to ascertain the risk of cross-species contamination of humans from infected cattle or sheep.

Even more serious is the belief that, according to Dr. Richard F. Marsh, a veterinarian at the University of Wisconsin in Madison, mad cow disease may have risen spontaneously in American cattle, without them receiving any tainted feed at all![181]

According to Dr. Joseph Gibbs, a leading mad cow disease expert at the National Insti-

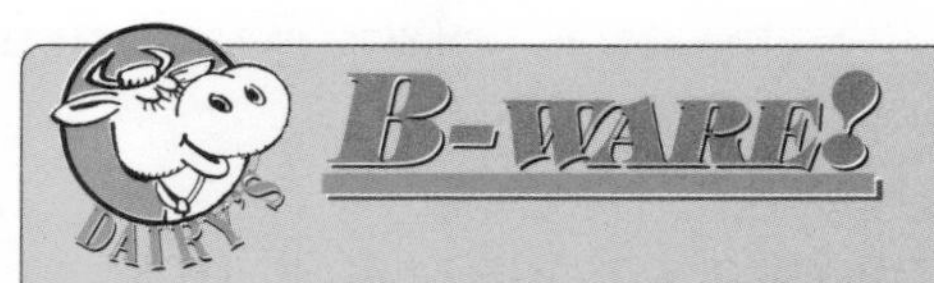

Many milk users warn, "Beware! If you don't drink milk, where will you get your vitamin B-12?" That's a good question— if you don't use *any* animal products. You need B-12 for maintaining healthy blood and nerves. The recommended daily allowance is just 2 micrograms, but some experts believe that only 1 microgram is necessary[A].

So, where can you find B-12 besides milk and meat? *Better Than Milk?*, a soy product by Sovex Natural Foods, is fortified with vitamin B-12, as are many other milk alternatives, cereals, and certain brands of nutritional yeast flakes. A product has B-12 if the word "cyanocobalamin" is on the label. Most multivitamin tablets also contain B-12. New research is showing that organically grown vegetables may also be a good source.[B] But don't overdo it. Your body can store a several-year supply[C] of B-12, and your actual need is very low. So don't B worried. Just B smart!

A: Am J Clin Nutr 1988;48:852-58
B: Plant and Soil 1994;167:305-311
C: The Power of Your Plate, p. 184

Substituting just 20 grams of soy protein for animal protein daily can "significantly lower serum concentrations of total cholesterol, LDL cholesterol, and triglycerides."

(The volunteers in this study consumed the same amounts of fat and cholesterol, regardless of which protein they were eating. Study author James Anderson, MD, concluded that "Soy...is grossly underused by the American public."

New England Journal of Medicine 1995;333(5):276-82

tute of Neurological Disorders and Stroke in Bethesda, MD, spontaneous cases of mad cow disease may occur in one cow in every million each year.[181] Such a cow contracts the disease naturally, without any exposure to other forms of the disease in its feed or in its herd.

With 150 million cows in the US, that means that 150 could develop mad cow disease each year all on their own, even without being exposed to tainted feed.[181] How many of those cows would be rendered and fed to other cows or other animals? No one knows.

In considering the milk consumption issue, perhaps milk author Frank Oski, MD, sums up the subject best:

"The slogan goes, 'Milk has something for everybody.' Who can argue with that? Of course, that 'something' might be diarrhea, iron-deficiency anemia, or even a heart attack!"[182]

How Now Soy Cow?

No wonder many people are eliminating cow's milk from their diet and are learning to milk *soy cows* or *tofu cows* instead. They're finding that *rice cows* and *oat cows* give udderly wonderful milk, too!

The phytoestrogens in soy beans and unrefined soy products are natural inhibitors for several types of cancer.[183] Soy may also boost the body's immunities when combined with low caloric intake.[184]

There is much evidence suggesting that compounds present in soybeans can prevent cancer in many different organ systems.

"QUOTE"

Journal of Nutrition 1995;125(3 Suppl):733S-743S

Soybeans contain relatively high concentrations of several compounds with "demonstrated anticarcinogenic activity."

Journal of the American Dietetic Association 1991;91(7):836-840

For those who want to stay young at heart, soy protein may aid in lowering blood pressure and have an anti-atherogenic (prevents plaque build up) effect in the system.[185] Whether refined soy protein offers as much protection as the whole soy bean is being studied, but some researchers feel that it may be comparable.

Moooove Over Milk?

For those who are concerned about their bones, one team of investigators reported that "Soybean milk is an excellent source for increasing bone mineral density and mechanical bone strength...the peptides (proteins) in the soybean milk are effective for the acceleration of intestinal calcium absorption."[186]

Even those who are unable to use soy protein don't have to despair. There are many different kinds of delicious, wholesome grain or nut milks that can be made at home or purchased at most health food stores.

But milk, whether animal or vegetable, is not essential for adult nutrition. A diet rich in grains, fruits, vegetables, and legumes will supply the nutritional elements you need to have vibrant health—including B-12, which is available in many non-animal foods and supplements.

But, if you want "milk," there are many recipes for great homemade milks. (See page 125.) And **Sovex Natural Foods** has excellent soy milks, yogurt, and ice cream! Most are B-12 enriched and casein-free. They also have non-soy dairy substitutes for soy-sensitive individuals. They're the ***cream of the crop***!

Such homemade or store bought substitutes will make the transition from cow's milk much easier. But, the choice is still yours to

Soy milk, compared to cow's milk, "induced significant reductions" in triglycerides and LDL-cholesterol, as well as a "significant increase" in HDL-cholesterol levels.

J of the American College of Nutrition 1992;11 Suppl;69S-73S

make. And that's why this book was written, to help you make a more informed decision on this important subject.

In weighing the evidence, consider these words from milk researchers: "Cow's milk may be an unfortunate substitute for human milk in infancy or a risky food source thereafter, or both."[187]

So, go ahead and keep that car in your garage. Use the VCR to view all the ***Let's Eat!*** videos, including ***MOOOOve Over Milk!*** Don't forget to return the calls on your answering machine, and enjoy your microwave popcorn (without the butter, of course!)

But the milk in the fridge? Well, perhaps it's ***moooo***ving time!

"Perhaps when the public is educated as to the hazards of milk, only calves will be left to drink the real thing."

Don't Drink Your Milk, p. 100

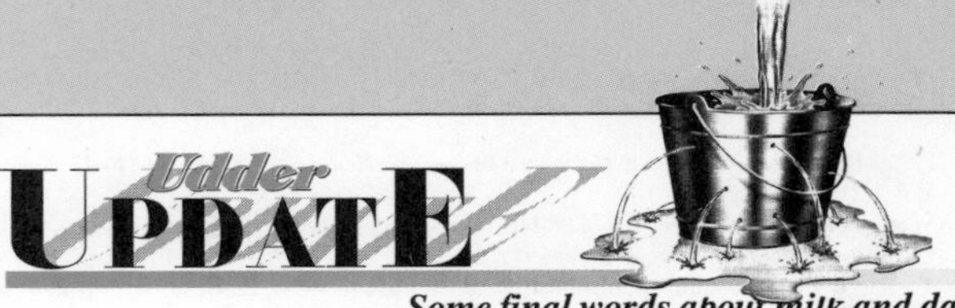

Some final words about milk and dairy

Does "the milk is necessary" argument bucket have a few holes? You've seen quite a bit of evidence, but here is a sampling of some of the information we didn't have room to fit anywhere else in this publication—and there was alot!

- **"In certain countries a particularly high or low frequency of ischemic heart disease is paralleled by milk consumption. Finland has the highest coronary mortality rate for middle-aged men...in the World Health Organization study of 21 areas. The consumption data show that Finland has the highest per capita intake of total milk and whole milk."**
  - *British J of Preventive and Social Medicine 1977;31:81-85*

- **In several countries, a "high positive correlation" was found between the per capita consumption of dairy products and the risk of juvenile diabetes.**
  - *American J of Clincial Nutrition 1990;51(3):489-491*

- **"Foods which are ingested frequently, and cow's milk in particular, are a common cause of delayed-in-onset allergy."**
  - *Journal of Family Practice 1979;9(2):223-232*

- **"IGF-1 enhanced the growth of human pancreatic cancer cells." (IGF-1 may be present in the milk of rBGH-treated cows)**
  - *Cancer Research 1995;55(10):2007-2011*

- **"Because of the concentration of organochlorine compounds (DDT, polychlorinated biphenyls, hexacholorobenzene, hexacholorocyclohexane, etc.) in fat, their accumulation is particularly high in the milk gland and leads to elevated concentrations in the colostrum and milk produced...These concentrated compounds are ultimately passed to both human and animal newborns and infants."**
  - *Archives of Toxicology 1985;56(3):195-200*

- **Recent studies "provide further evidence that BSE agent has been transmitted to man," causing the new variant CJD in humans.**
  - *Nature 1996;383:666-667*

REFERENCES

1. Proceedings of the Society for Experimental Biology and Medicine 1990 Nov;193:143-159; Epidemiology 1994 May;5(3):324-331.
2. Swaisgood, HE. Characteristics of edible fluids of animal origin: milk. In: Fennema OR, Ed. Food Chemistry, New York: Marcel Dekker, 1985.
3. Motil, KJ. Breast-feeding: public health and clinical overviews. In: Grand RJ, Sutphen JL Dietz, WH, Eds. Pediatric Nutrition. Boston: Butterworths, 1987.
4. American Journal of Clinical Nutrition 1990;51(1):37-46
5. Pediatrics 1981;68:394-397; Journal of Pediatrics 1981;98:540; Nutrition and the MD 1983 May.
6. Pediatrics 1992;89(6):1105-1109; American Journal of Clinical Nutrition 1993;58:343-348; Journal of Pediatriatic Gastroenterology and Nutrition 1993;16(1):1-3.
7. Journal of the American Dietetic Association 1994;94(3):314-316; Diabetes1996;45:178-182; Lancet 1996;348(9032):905-906, 926-928.
8. Diabetes Care 1994 Jan;17(1):13-19; Nutrition Abstracts and Reviews 1995 Jan;65(1):107.
9. New England Journal of Medicine 1992 July;327(5):302-307.
10. Medical Tribune 1992 Aug;33(16):2.
11. Diabetes Care 1994 Dec;17(12):1488-1490.
12. Diabetes 1993 Dec;42:1786-1789.
13. The New England Journal of Medicine 1992 Jul;327(5):348-349.
14. American Journal of Clinical Nutrition 1976 Jul;29:689-690.
15. Chaney, MS and Ross, ML. Nutrition (7th ed.). Boston: Houghton Mifflin Company, 1966, p. 383.
16. Diehl HA. Dynamic Living, p. 58.
17. Journal of Pediatrics 1995 Jan;126(1):34-39; J Allergy and Clinical Immunology 1994;93(1):193; Pediatric News 9(6):56-57; Lancet 1978;1(8059):304-305.
18. Clinical Trends in Family Practice 1978 Sept-Oct.
19. Allergy 1994;49:295-298; P-N 1982 Nov/Dec;23-30.
20. Journal of Family Practice 1979;9(2):223-232.
21. Pediatrics 1976;57(5):675-680.
22. Nutrition Abstracts and Reviews (Series A) 1994;64(3):270
23. Postgraduate Medicine 1994;95(1):113-120; Israel Journal of Medical Sciences 1979;15:369-373.
24. American Journal of Gastroenterology 1993;88(9):476; Digestive Diseases and Sciences 1995 Jul; 40(7):1506-1510; Medical Tribune for the Family Physician 1993 Nov;34(21).
25. Journal of Nutrition 1993;123(8):1370-1376; Dynamic Nutrition Research 1993;3:40-51.
26. Circulation 1993 Dec;88(6):2771-2779.
27. International Journal of Cardiology 1994;46(3):197-207.
28. Atherosclerosis 1989;76(1):55-61
29. Diehl, HA. To Your Health, Lifestyle Medicine Institute. Loma Linda, CA 1987, pp. 48-49.
30. Journal of Clinical Biochemistry and Nutrition 1990;9(1):61-66.
31. Gibney, M. *Animal and Vegetable Proteins in Lipid Metabolism and Atherosclerosis*, Alan R. Liss, Inc, New York; 1983. (Chapter) Studies on the Use of a Soybean Protein Diet for the Management of Human Hyperlipoproteinemias, Sirtori, CR, et al, pp. 135-148.
32. British Journal of Preventive and Social Medicine 1977;31:81-85.
33. McDougall, J. McDougall's Medicine, New Century Publishers, Piscataway, NJ, 1985, p. 62.
34. Journal of the American Medical Association (JAMA) 1984;252(6):799-802.
35. Calcified Tissue International 1992;50:14-18; American Journal of Clinical Nutrition 1972;25:518; Clinical Orthopaedics and Related Research 1980;152:55; Food Balance Sheets 1979-1981 average, Food And Agriculture Organization (FAO) of the United Nations, Rome, 1984; FAO Production Year - book 1984;37:263.
36. Journal of Clinical Investigation 1987;80:979-982.
37. JAMA 1984;252(6):799-802; Journal of Clinical Investigation 1975;56:311; British Medical Journal 1982;285:585.
38. American Journal of Clinical Nutrition 1972;25:518; Clinical Orthopaedics 1980;152:35; FAO Production Yearbook 1984;37:263.
39. American Journal of Clinical Nutrition 1987;46:685-687; American Journal of Clinical Nutrition 1991;53:132-142; Science 1986;233:519-520; Journal of Nutrition 1981;111:545, 553; Journal of Nutrition 1974;104(6):695-700; Journal of the American Dietetic Association 1980;76:148-151; Hospital Practice 1994 Nov 15;68.
40. Health 1993 September;28.
41. American Journal of Clinical Nutrition 1994 June;59(6):1356-1361.
42. American Journal of Clinical Nutrition 1995 April;61(4):909.
43. Nutrition Research 1994;14:19-20.
44. Journal of Nutrition 1986;116(7):1364-1370.
45. American Journal of Diseases of Children 1990;144:1159-1163; American Journal of Clinical Nutrition 1978;31:720(Abstract); Journal of Epidemiology and Community Health 1978;32:147-154; Journal of the American Dietetic Association 1978;72:264-270; Journal of the American Dietetic Association 1980;77:434-437; Pediatrics 1974;58:737-741.
46. National Research Council. Recommended Dietary Allowances. 10th Ed. Washington, DC: National Academy Press; 1989.

47. Messina, M and J, *The Dietician's Guide to Vegetarian Diets*, Aspen Publishers, Gaithersburg, MD, 1996, p. 83.
48. US Department of Agriculture. *Nationwide Food Consumption Survey 1977-1978. Food Intakes: Individuals in 48 States.* Year 1977-1978 (report 1-1). Hyattsville, MD: Consumer Nutrition Division; 1983. US Department of Agriculture. *Nationwide Food Consumption Survey. Continuing Survey of Food Intakes by Individuals. Men 19-50 Years, 1 Day, 1985* (report 85-3). Hyattsville, MD; 1986. US Department of Agriculture. *Nationwide Food Consumption Survey. Continuing Survey of Food Intakes by Individuals. Women 19-50 Years and Their Children 1-5 Years, 4 Days, 1985* (report 85-4); Hyattsville, MD;1987.
49. FASEB Journal 1987 1:394-97; Nutrition Today 1988 Jan-Feb;4-7.
50. Journal of Nutrition 1981;111(3):545-552.
51. British Journal of Urology 1982 Dec;54(6):590-593.
52. American J of Clinical Nutrition 1968;21(9):898-903; Nutrition and Metabolism 1974;16:1-9.
53. Journal of the American Dietetic Association 1985 Jul;85(7):841-845.
54. Journal of Nutrition 1990 Jan;120(1):134-136.
55. American Journal of Clinical Nutrition 1994 Jun;59(6):1356-1361.
56. Calcified Tissue International 1992;50:14-18.
57. Journal of the American Medical Association 1992 Nov;268(17):2403-2408.
58. American Journal of Clinical Nutrition 1993 58:398-406; American Journal of Clinical Nutrition 1979 Apr;32(4):741-749.
59. Messina, M and J, *The Dietician's Guide to Vegetarian Diets*, Aspen Publishers, Gaithersburg, MD, 1996, p. 92.
60. Journal of the American Dietetic Association 1988;88:352-355.
61. Nutrition Reviews 1970;28:223-226.
62. American Journal of Clinical Nutrition 1968;21(8):827-835.
63. Food and Agricultural Organization (FAO). Rice: Grain for Life, World Food Problems. Rome, Italy, 1966; American Journal of Clinical Nutrition 1971;24(3):318-323, 324-328.
64. Pediatric Research 1992;31(5):524-527.
65. American Journal of Clinical Nutrition 1990;51(4):656-657.
66. Committee on Diet, Nutrition, and Cancer of the National Research Council. 1982.
67. Cancer Letters 1996;104:129-132.
68. Journal of the National Cancer Institute 1989;81(4):278-286.
69. Nutrition Report International 1982;26:793-806; Cancer Research 1986;46:4395-4399; Journal of Nutrition 1974;104:1586-1583.
70. British Journal of Cancer 1978;37:974-982.
71. Cancer 1979 May;43(5):2125; Regulatory Toxicology and Pharmacology 1986;6(1):24-54; International Journal of Cancer 1991 Sept; 49(2):161-167.
72. Nutrition and Cancer 1989;12(4):333-341; Cancer Causes and Control 1994;5:422-432.
73. Lancet 1976 Nov;2(7996):1184-1186.
74. British Journal of Cancer 1990 Mar;61(3):456-459; Nutrition and Cancer 1989;12(4):333-341.
75. Nutrition and Cancer 1990;13(1-2):89-99.
76. International Journal of Cancer 1989;43:608-612.
77. Revista de Sandiad e Higiene Publica 1994;68(3):361-376.
78. Lancet 1989 July;2(8654):66-71; Cancer 1994;74(4):1309-1317; Am J Epidemiol 1989;130(5):904-910
79. Lancet 1989 July;2(8654):66-71.
80. British Journal of Cancer 1989;59(1):92-96.
81. Messina, M and J, *The Dietician's Guide to Vegetarian Diets*, Aspen Publishers, Gaithersburg, MD, 1996, p. 177.
82. Journal of Pediatrics 1985;107(3):372-376.
83. New England Journal of Medicine 1992;326(18):1213-1215.
84. American Journal of Clinical Nutrition 1994;60(4):619-630.
85. Canadian Medical Association Journal 1992;147(9):1308, 1313; Nephron 1987;47(1):78-80.
86. Department of Health and Human Services. Grade "A" pasteurized milk ordinance. 21 CFR 131.110, 1989, 243.
87. Pediatrics 1963;31:512-525.
88. New England Journal of Medicine 1992;326(18):1173-1177.
89. Proceedings of the Royal Society of Medicine 1952;45:401; Principles and Practice of Endocrinology and Metabolism. Philadelphia, PA: Lippincott; 1990:417-423.
90. Leukemia Research 1985;9(6):709-711; Your Good Health 1994 Jan/Feb;10.
91. American Journal of Epidemiology 1980;112(1):80-92.
92. Bibliotheca Haematologica 1970;36:649-653.
93. Journal of the American Medical Association 1975;232(13):1333-1336.
94. Journal of the National Cancer Institute 1981;66(6):1027-1030.
95. American Journal of Epidemiology 1980;112(1):80-92.
96. Public Health Service, Centers for Disease Control, Atlanta, GA. EPI-770-36-2, January 8, 1979.
97. The Bovine Practitioner 1979 Nov;14:115-120.
98. American Journal of Industrial Medicine 1988;14(1):63-72.
99. Hoard's Dairyman 1992 August;25:571.

100. Journal of the American Veterinary Medical Association 1981 Oct;179(7):704-707.
101. Vegetarian Voice 1995;21(2):13.
102. Miller, J. Update on Federal Condemnation for Lymphosarcoma in U.S. Cattle, Proceedings of the United States Animal Husbandry Association Meeting, October 29, 1991; Journal of the National Cancer Institute 1985 Mar;74(3):711-714.
103. Sorenson, DK Prevalence and Economics of Bovine Leukosis in the United States, Bovine Leukosis Symposium, May 22-23, 1979; The Wall Street Journal. May 31, 1991.
104. Japanese Journal of Cancer Research 1993 Mar;84(3):inside front cover.
105. Israel Journal of Medical Sciences 1994;30(5-6):387-391.
106. Neuroepidemiology 1993;12(1):15-27; 1993;12(4):234-240; 1992;11(4-6):304-312; Medical Hypotheses 1992;39(3):275-280; Acta Neurologica Scandinavica 1990;81(3):223-228; Acta Neurologica Scandinavica 1992;86(1):91-94;1993;88:190-198.
107. Neuroepidemiology 1992;11(4-6):304-312.
108. Neuroepidemiology 1993;12(1):15-27.
109. Rubino, MJ. Inactivation of Bovine Leukemia Virus in Milk. Thesis, University of Iowa, December, 1980; American Journal of Epidemiology 1980;112(1):80-92.
110. Journal of the National Cancer Institute 1981 November;67(5):1157-1163; Miller, JM. The Biology of Bovine Leukemia Virus Infection in Cattle, reprinted from Viruses in Naturally Occurring Cancers, Cold Springs Harbor Conferences on Cell Proliferation, Vol. 7, 1980, Cold Springs Harbor Laboratory, pp. 901-909.
111. Lancet 1974;2(871):30-31; Journal of the National Cancer Institute 1972;49(5):1463-1467.
112. Advances in Cancer Research 1978;28:251-311.
113. Leukemia Research 1984;8(3):315-321.
114. Journal of Health and Healing 15(4):3-7; Journal of Clinical Microbiology 1992;30(1):185-191.
115. Advances in Cancer Research 1978;28:251-311; Journal of the National Cancer Institute 1977;59(3):851-853; Canadian Journal of Comparative Medicine 1979;43(2):173-179; The Bovine Practitioner 1979;14:115-120; Bibliotheca Haematologica 1975 Oct;43:232-234; Science 1981;213(4511):1014-1016.
116. Sorensen, DK. Clinical Manifestation of Bovine Leukosis Symposium, 1979, USDA.
117. American Journal of Veterinary Research 1995 Apr;56(4):445-449.
118. Veterinary Microbiology 1994 Nov;42(2-3):181-189.
119. Journal of Health and Healing 15(4):3-7.
120. Lancet 1974;2(871):30-31; Cancer Research 1974;34(10):2745-2757.
121. Canadian Journal of Veterinary Research 1992 Oct;56(4):353-359.
122. Journal of Food Protection 1990;53:441-452.
123. Journal of Dairy Science 1992;75:2327-2343.
124. Biggs, T. Milk, Cheese, and Whey—Why Not? College Press, Collegedale, TN, 1976, p. 11.
125. Advances in Cheese Technology, 1958, FAO, United Nations, p. 73.
126. Journal of Dairy Science 1992;75(9):2330.
127. American Journal of Epidemiology 1980 Feb;111(2):247-253.
128. CDC 1985, Milk-borne Salmonellosis—Illinois, Weekly Report; 34:200; CDC 1985, Milk-borne Salmonellosis—Illinois, Update;34:215; FDA Consumer 1986;20:18; Journal of Food Protection 1981;44:381.
129. Journal of Food Protection 1984;47:20; Journal of Food Protection 1985;48:1062.
130. New England Journal of Medicine 1996 May;334(20):1281-1286.
131. Journal of Dairy Science 1988 April;71:2809-2816.
132. Journal of the American Medical Association 1992 Dec;268(22):3203-3207; Journal of Milk Food Technology 1970;33:280.
133. Committee on Diet, Nutrition and Cancer. National Academy Press, Washington DC, 1982.
134. Science 1981 Aug;213(4511):1014-1016; Bovine Lymphosarcoma. The Compendium on Continuing Education for the Practicing Veterinarian 1980;2(11):235-242.
135. Annals of the Rheumatic Diseases 1994 Jul;53(7):481.
136. The Palm Beach Post, Oct. 30, 1994.
137. Journal of the American Medical Association 1992 Dec;268(22):3203-3207.
138. Reviews of Infectious Diseases 1988;10:111-124.
139. New England Journal of Medicine 1996 May;334(20):1324-1325.
140. Food Technology 1969;23:1178; Journal of the American Veterinary Medical Association 1966;149:1079.
141. Journal of Dairy Science 1988 Apr;71:2809-2816.
142. Clinical Pathology 1993;46:1057-1058.
143. New England Journal of Medicine 1985 Feb;312(7);404-407.
144. New England Journal of Medicine 1988 Sep;29:319(13):823-828.
145. New England Journal of Medicine 1985 Feb;312(7):438-440.
146. Bryan FL. Listeria monocytogenes. In: Riemann H, Bryan FLl, eds. Food-borne infections and intoxications. 2nd ed. New York: Academic Press, 1979:266-268.
147. Epidemiology and Infection 1990;104:345-350.
148. Dorland's Illustrated Medical Dictionary 28th ed. W.B. Saunders Co Philadelphia 1994.
149. Journal of Dairy Science 1992;75(9):2327-2343; Epidemiology and Infection 1993;111:181-187.
150. Internal Medicine News and Cardiology News 1994 Nov;27(22):7.

151. Microbiological Pathology 1994 Jun;16(6):401-411.
152. Hoard's Dairyman, January 25, 1995, p. 43.
153. Journal of Infectious Disease 1994 Feb;169(2):449-451.
154. Veterinary Record 1981;109(24):532-533; Journal of Clinical Microbiology 1992;30(1):166-171.
155. Hoard's Dairyman, January 25, 1993, p. 43; Paratuberculosis and Crohn's Disease: A Relationship? Dr. Michael Collins, School of Veterinary Medicine, U of Wisconsin (paper)
156. Clinical Microbiol Review 1994 Jul;7(3):328-345; J of Clinical Microbiology 1993;31(5):1241-1245.
157. Gut 1992 Jul;33(7):890-896.
158. Journal of the American Veterinary Association 1994 Feb 15;204(4):636-641.
159. Food and Drug Administration publication number 229.
160. Your Health June 1994.
161. AP Online February 1994.
162. Daily News, AP, Aug. 6, 1992.
163. Atlanta Journal, Jan 9, 1990; Journal of Environmental Pathology, Toxicology, and Oncology 1990 May/June;10(3)99-102; Environmental Contamination and Toxicology 1991;47:817-21.
164. Consumer Reports 1992 May:330-332; Delicious, December 1995, p. 9.
165. Cancer Research 1995 June;55:2463-2469.
166. Scientific American 1995 Jan;272(1):48-51, 54-57.
167. Veterinary Record 1991;128:199-203.
168. Reuters News Service report, November 25, 1995.
169. In These Times 1993 May 31;12-15.
170. In These Times 1993 May 17;12-13.
171. Annals of the New York Academy of Sciences 1994;724:246-258.
172. Science 1996 Aug;273(5275):622-626.
173. Reuters News Service August 1, 1996.
174. Reuters News Service August 1, 1996.
175. Reuters News Service August 19, 1996.
176. Lancet 1995;346:1208-1210.
177. Journal of Infectious Disease 1990 Mar;161(3):467-472.
178. Journal of the American Veterinary Association
179. Journal of General Virology 1991 Mar;72(Pt 3):589-584.
180. Hulse, V. Milk Gate, Marble Mountain Publishing, Phoenix, OR, 1996, p. 32.
181. New York Times News Service, 3/11/97
182. Oski, F. Don't Drink Your Milk, p. 81.
183. Journal of the American Dietetic Association 1991;91(7):836-840; Chemotherapy1994;40(4):272-278; Nutrition and Cancer 1994;21(2):113-131; Cancer Investigation 1996;14(6):597-608; European Urology 1996;30(2):243-248; Journal of Nutrition 1995;125(3 Suppl):567S-569S; 698S-708S;757S-770S;717S-724S;735-743S;777S-783S; Cancer Letters 1994;78(1-3):151-157; Obstetrics and Gynecology 1996;87(5 pt 2):897-904; Maturitas 1995;22(3):167-175; Proceedings of the Society for Experimental Biology and Medicine 1995;208(1):124-130; Nutrition and Cancer 1995;23(3):259-270.
184. Cancer Letters 1994 78:151-7.
185. Nutrition Abstracts and Reviews (Series A) 1994 64(2); 65(2).
186. American Institute of Nutrition 1993 "Dietary Soybean Protein Compared with Casein Retards Senescence in the Senescence Accelerated Mouse."; Journal of Nutrition, Science, and Vitaminology 1994;40:201-211.
187. Lancet 1974;213:1014.

"Epidemiologic studies have not provided evidence that high dairy product consumption by adults prevents fractures; in fact, the results of several studies suggest positive associations." (In other words, milk-drinking may actually increase the risk of fractures).

American J of Clinical Nutrition
1995;61(6 Suppl):1407S-1415S

The Missing Link...

Some scientists study primates, trying to find information about evolution's "missing link." Other scientists studying chimps have found a possible missing link in the evolution of certain killer diseases in man—diseases that could be passed through milk.

Bois and Roger, two baby chimps, were fed unpasteurized milk from a cow whose milk was "an abundant and constant" source of bovine leukemia virus (BLV). Both chimps died in less than a year of erythroleukemia and Pneumocystis carinii pneumonia—the latter being a hallmark of AIDS infections.

Cancer Research 1974;34(10):2745-2757

While milk and dairy may have been safe foods in the past, earth's growing pollution problem and the widespread inhumane treatment of animals have made them questionable food sources today.

But don't worry! Our incredibly efficient bodies were designed by an incredibly efficient, loving Creator who knows what we need to enjoy maximum health and vitality! Because He knows how we work, God knows what we need to work best and where to find it! He promises you that with His ***Designer Diet***, He will

"Satisfy your mouth with good things; so that your youth is renewed like the eagles."

Psalm 103:5

What "good things" will renew your youth? The ***Designer Diet*** origianlly given to humans: Fruits, nuts, grains, legumes, and vegetables. Milks made from plant sources taste wonderful, are very satisfying and nutritious, and are free from hormones, antibiotics, and possible diseases.

Many today are choosing a dairy-free diet as an economic and healthy lifestyle choice. Such a change takes care, planning, and effort, but He who created the *Designer Diet* can re-create a desire in us for that diet! Questions? We look forward to hearing from you.

Come and Get it! RECIPES!

Some of the best cholesterol-free cooking you'll ever find is waiting for you on each of the ***Let's Eat!*** video programs. The recipes are easy to fix, easy on your budget, and even easier to eat!

The ***Let's Eat!*** program ***MOOOOve Over Milk*** will show you how to make some of the cream of the crop dairy replacement recipes—that don't skim off any taste. These delicious recipes will help you put milk out to pasture without stalling—and without any bum steers.

Let's Eat! Come and get it! But while you're waiting to get your video, try these favorites of Dr. Vicki Griffin, radio commentator, health author, and ***Let's Eat!*** host.

Tropical Rice Milk

- ❑ **1 C .... Well-cooked brown rice**
- ❑ **2/3 C ..... Raw cashews**
- ❑ **1/3 C ..... Unsweetened coconut**
- ❑ **1 Tb ...... Vanilla**
- ❑ **1 tsp ...... Salt**
- ❑ **2-3 Tb ... Honey**

- *Grind cashews and coconut in blender.*
- *Add all ingredients and blend in 3 C water until very frothy and creamy.*
- *Pour into 1/2 gallon container, add water to fill; shake well before using.*
- *Pour through a strainer to get a smoother milk.*
- *For richer, sweeter milk, add less water.*
- *Add very little water for a thick cream to pour over fruit.*
- *For use in mashed potatoes or gravy, omit vanilla and honey.*

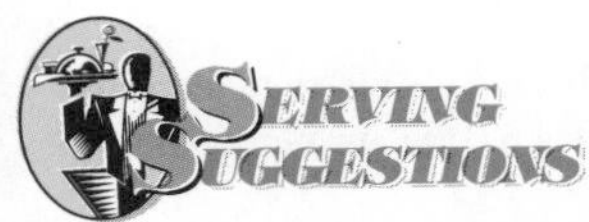

1. **Great over any hot or dry cereal—especially granola!**
2. **Use to replace 1/2 of water to make creamier hot cereals.**
3. **Pour over toast and bananas, topped with raisins; or over steamed rice.**

FOR MORE FREE DAIRY-FREE RECIPES, CHECK BOX ON PAGE 144.

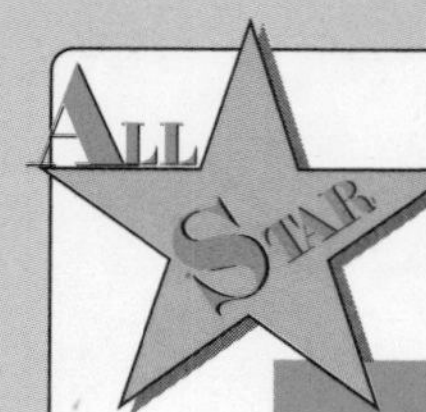

American Cheese

An MVP for your taste-tempting team!

- ❑ 1/2 C .... Pimento
- ❑ 1/2 C .... Unbleached, white flour
- ❑ 1/2 C .... Nutritional yeast flakes[A]
- ❑ 1 C .... Water
- ❑ 1/6 C .... Sesame tahini[B]
- ❑ 2 Tb .... Lemon juice
- ❑ 1 1/2 tsp .... Salt

- ★ *Blend all ingredients **thoroughly** in blender.*
- ★ *Pour into a small, coated bread pan.*
- ★ *Bake at 350º for 30 minutes, or until firm-looking in the center.*
- ★ *It will settle and firm as it cools.*
- ★ *Refrigerate.*
- ★ *When cold, run knife around outer edges and turn cheese out onto a serving plate.*
- ★ *Slice before serving.*

A. Available at most health food stores
B. Not the same as sesame butter; available at most health food stores.

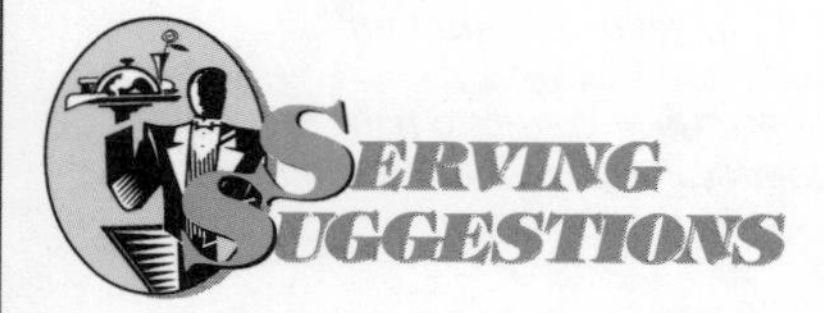

1. This is my son's favorite cheese. He (and we!) loves to put it into steamed corn tortillas with shredded lettuce and Marvi-whip mayonnaise (recipe on p. 128).
2. Try this cheese in sandwiches or on crackers.
3. Sometimes I bake this cheese with 1/2 C sliced olives for a special treat. It's incredible!

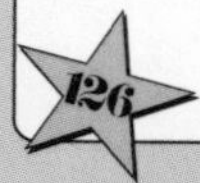

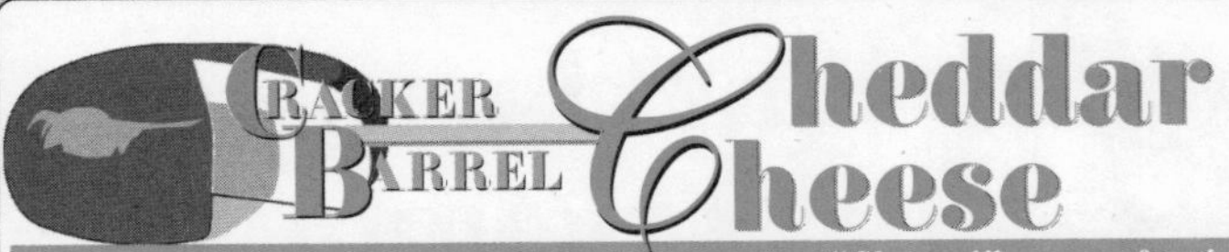

Take one taste, and you'll be saying "Cheese!" more often!

- ❑ 1/2 C .... Sesame tahini[A]
- ❑ 1/4 C .... Lemon juice
- ❑ 4 Tb .... Nutritional yeast flakes[B]
- ❑ 4 oz .... Pimento
- ❑ 1 1/2 tsp .... Salt
- ❑ 1 tsp .... Onion powder
- ❑ 1/2 tsp .... Garlic powder
- ❑ 3 Tb .... Unflavored Emes gelatin[B] (dissolved in 1/2 C cold water)

- *Bring an additional 1/2 C water to boil.*
- *Place ALL ingredients, including dissolved. Emes and 1/2 C boiling water into a blender.*
- *Blend* ***very thoroughly****, until smooth and creamy.*
- *Pour into a mold (A small bread pan works very well as a mold.)*
- *Chill until thoroughly set: at least 3 hours.*
- *Turn out of pan onto dish. Slices and melts nicely.*

A. Not the same as sesame butter; available at most health food stores.
B. Available at most health food stores

1. This cheese is delicious melted on toast, veggies, noodles, or rice.
2. A little over steaming black beans or chile beans is a real treat!
3. Use it in sandwiches or tortillas.
4. It is delicious frozen, then grated on pizza, enchiladas, manicotti, or casseroles. This will be one of your favorites!

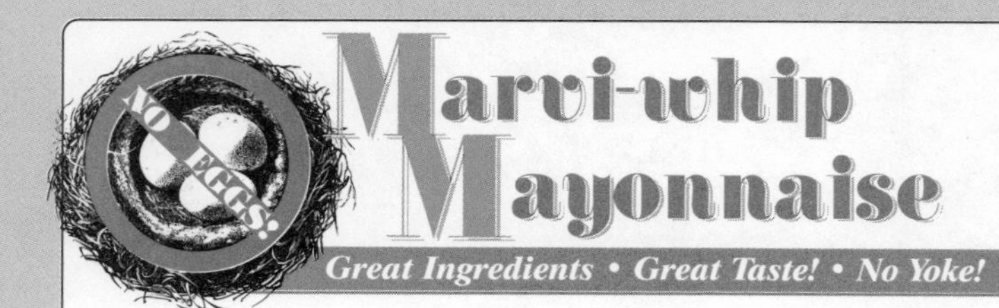

- 2 C .... Soft tofu
- 1 Tb .... Nutritional yeast flakes
- 1 tsp .... Salt
- 1/4 C .... Lemon juice
- 1/3 C .... Water (or just enough to blend contents smoothly
- 1 tsp .... Onion powder
- 1/2 tsp .... Garlic powder
- 1/2 C .... Olive oil

OR

- 1/3 C .... RAW cashews

- *Blend all ingredients **thoroughly** in blender.*
- *Chill and serve.*
- *For Italian dressing, add 1/2 tsp EACH:*
  - *Dill weed*
  - *Basil*
  - *Italian seasoning*

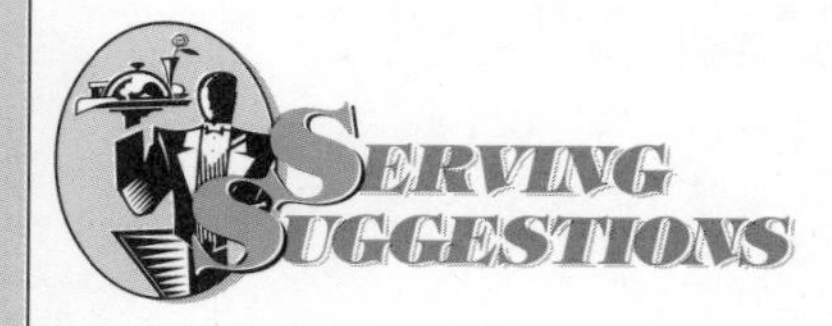

1. This delightful, light mayonnaise is delicious on salads or as a dip for raw veggies. You can also pour it over steamed asparagus, cabbage, or broccoli. Try it as a dip for steamed artichokes!
2. Put it on Mexican beans, haystacks, or as a taste-tempting topping over baked potatoes, spinkled with dill and chopped onions.
3. Use it as a sandwich spread or as a filling in pita bread. It's great as a topping for many savory casseroles, such as those made from rice, lentils, or garbanzo beans.
4. My husband loves it on his home-baked French fries—even in his soup! It's not hard to love this recipe! And it's good for you, too!!!

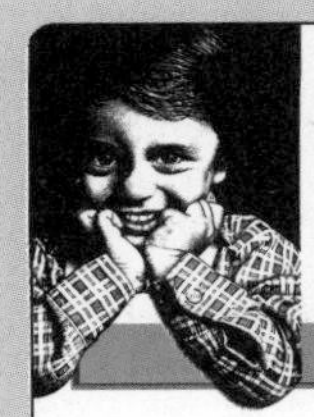

Dreamy Cream Whip

It's love at first bite!

- ❑ 2 C .... Soft tofu
- ❑ 1/2 C .... Canola oil
- ❑ 2 Tb .... Vanilla
- ❑ 2/3 C .... Honey
- ❑ Pinch .... Salt

*Blend ALL ingredients **thoroughly** in blender.*

Add SMALL amounts of water if necessary while blending to keep mixture moving in blender.

Chill and serve.

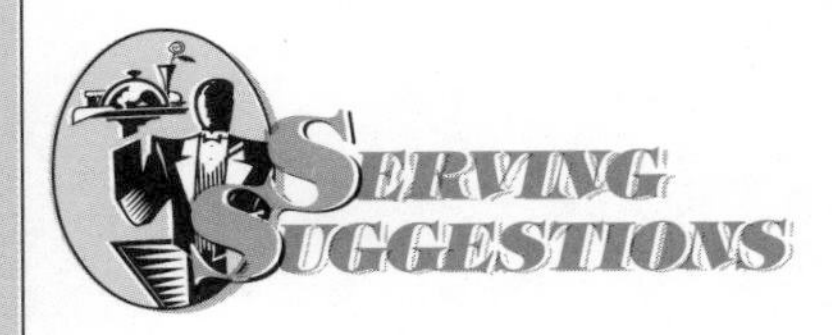

1. **This whipped treat is for special occasions and is superb on any pie, spooned on top of fruit salad cups, or even on a bowl of piping hot multi-grain cereral for a creamy, dreamy treat!**
2. **Try it as the crowning touch on golden waffles (send for FREE recipe to address on last page) smothered with fresh, juicy strawberries. Or, use the waffles, strawberries, and cream whip to make a luscious, delicious strawberry shortcake. Just layer waffles, berries, and cream as high as you want. It's a tasty treat that can't be beat!**

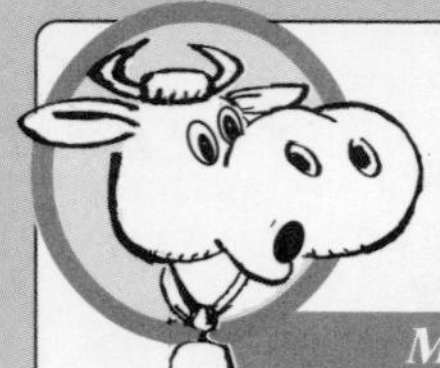

Better Butter

Much better than the udder butter!

- ❑ 1/2 C .... **Yellow cornmeal** (uncooked)
- ❑ 1/2 C .... **Shredded, unsweetened coconut**
- ❑ 1 tsp .... **Salt**
- ❑ 2 Tb .... **Nutritional yeast flakes**
- ❑ 1 tsp .... **Butter flavor**
- ❑ 2 C .... **Water**

- *Place cornmeal, coconut, and water in a small saucepan.*
- *Cover and simmer until cooked (20-30 minutes).*
- *Pour cooked contents into blender.*
- *Add all other ingredients PLUS 1/4 C more water.*
- *Blend until very creamy and smooth (usually takes several minutes).*
- *Pour into container and let cool (uncovered).*
- *Sets up very nicely when chilled in refrigerator.*

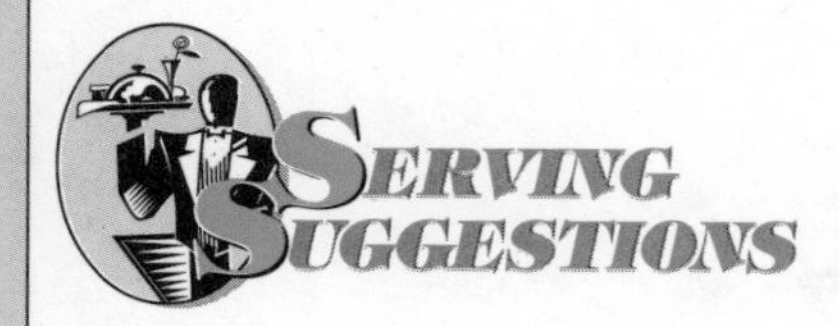

Serving Suggestions

1. For a "cheesy" flavor, add another 1 Tb nutritional yeast flakes.
2. For a grrrrreat garlic spread, add the extra nutitional yeast flakes PLUS a clove (or two!) of garlic.
3. For a delicious maple spread, omit the nutritional yeast and add 1 Tb of maple extract and 1/2 C honey. Talk about tasty toast!!
4. Better Butter is great on potatoes, bread, or veggies. You can even pour it, while it's hot, like hollandaise sauce over veggies. This is one of the most versatile spreads you'll ever make.
5. Try the maple version as a spread for waffles or as a hot sauce over steamed rice for breakfast. Top with raisins, granola, bananas—use your imagination! Make breakfast fun—and nutritious!

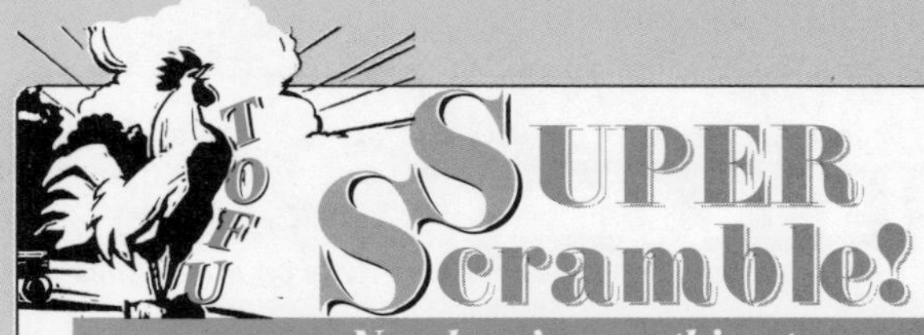

Tofu Super Scramble!

Now here's something to crow about!

Saute in a little water or olive oil in a large pan:

- ❑ 1 .... Medium diced onion
- ❑ 2-3 .... Garlic cloves, crushed

OR

- ❑ 1 1/2 tsp .... Garlic powder
- ❑ 2 pounds .... Firm tofu (drain, rinse, and crumble into small pieces into a skillet)

Stir in well:

- ❑ 2 Tb .... Chicken-like seasoning
- ❑ 4 Tb .... Nutritional yeast flakes
- ❑ 1/2 tsp .... Turmeric
- ❑ Salt (or Vege-sal) to taste

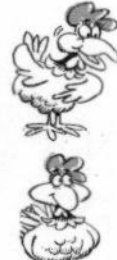

- *Cover and simmer for 10 minutes*
- *Then add 4 medium peeled, cubed, cooked potatoes (leftover baked potatoes work great!)*
- *Cover and simmer until flavors have blended*
- *Sprinkle with dry parsely to garnish*

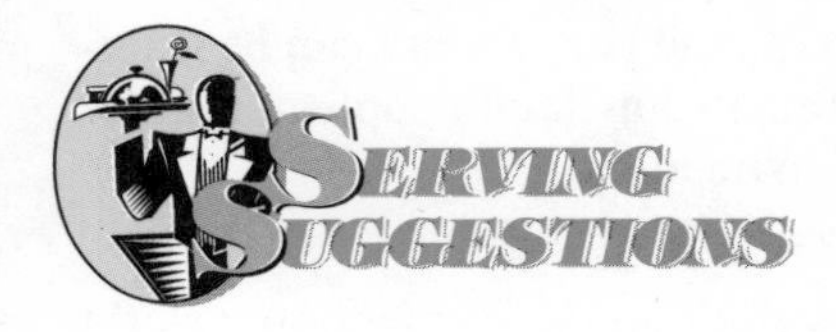

Serving Suggestions

1. My mouth is watering already! We love scrambled tofu in steamed tortillas with All Star American Cheese (p. 126), or with steamed broccoli or kale and a baked yam.
2. It is delicious cold in a pita pocket or in a whole wheat sandwich with sprouts and Marvi-whip Mayonnaise (p. 128), or served hot on toast.
3. For a zesty flair, try dicing 1/2 a green or red bell pepper and adding to the onion when you saute!
4. Try it cold for your next picnic, served on a bed of rice! You can also serve it with shredded cabbage and Totally French Dressing (write us for the recipe), and then...go hike!!!

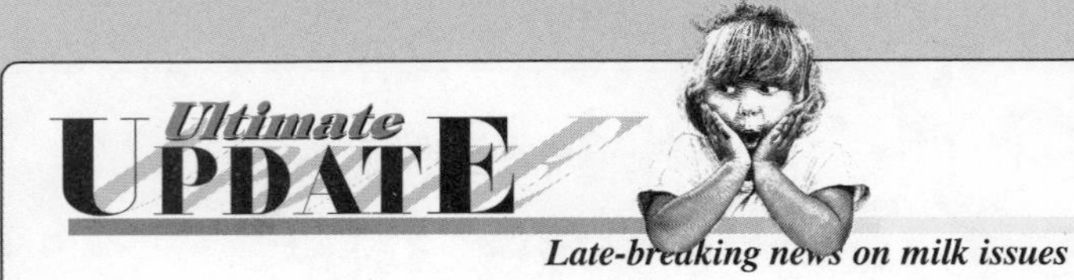

As we prepare to go to press, new studies on milk are making news almost daily. Here is a sampling of some of them.

- British scientists have reported the first direct evidence for a link between mad cow disease (BSE) and Creutzfeldt-Jakob Disease in humans. They warned that the "epidemic is in its early stages" and may not reach full scale for many years.

  ● United Press International, October 23, 1996

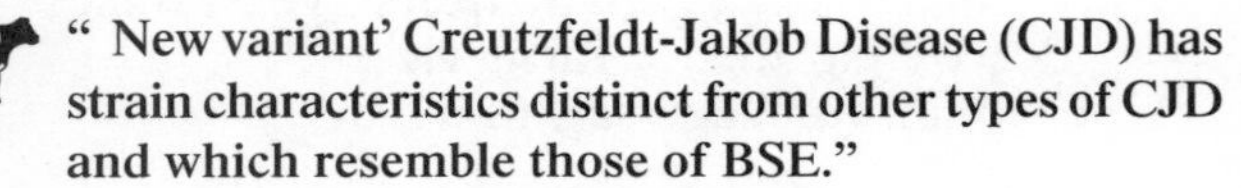

- " New variant' Creutzfeldt-Jakob Disease (CJD) has strain characteristics distinct from other types of CJD and which resemble those of BSE."

  ● Nature 1996;383(6602):685-690

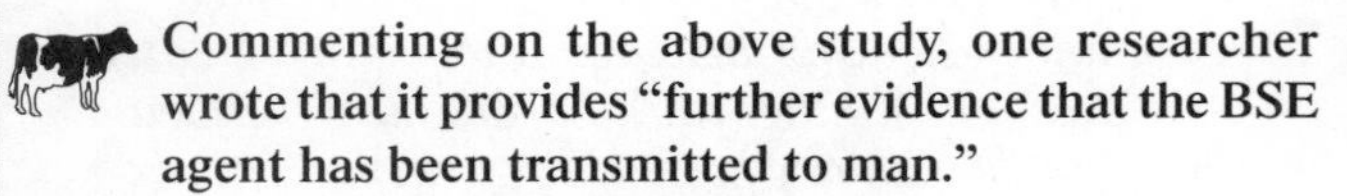

- Commenting on the above study, one researcher wrote that it provides "further evidence that the BSE agent has been transmitted to man."

  ● Nature 1996;383(6602):666-667

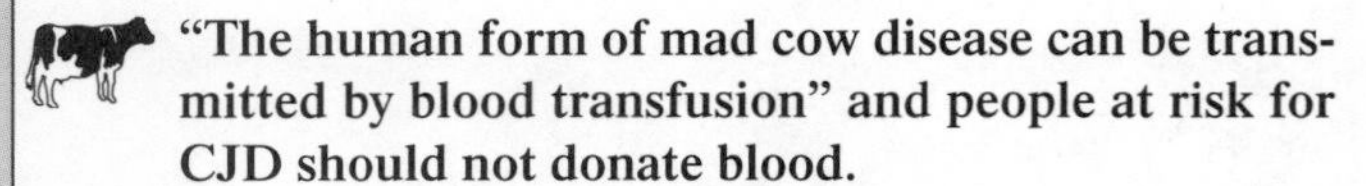

- "The human form of mad cow disease can be transmitted by blood transfusion" and people at risk for CJD should not donate blood.

  ● Reuters News Service, March 26, 1997

- Because of the possibility of BSE infection, gelatin has been removed from the Generally Recognized As Safe (GRAS) list by the FDA.

  ● Reuters News Service, April 25, 1997

- A golden retriever that died in Norway may have died of "mad dog" disease. Its brain resembled the brains of cows that die of BSE. It may have contracted the disease from dog food tainted with rendered beef infected with BSE.

  ● The Associated Press, April 21, 1997

YOU'VE GOT TO SEE THEM ALL!

The Let's Eat! video on milk is a fast-paced, eye-opening adventure into better health! One of the couuntry's leading pediatricians will update you on the latest information on dairy produts. Take a tour of a dairy farm and hear what workers have to say. Learn how to milk a "soy cow" and "say cheese" heatlhfully! It's 60-minutes of educational excitement! But the milk video is just one part of the Let's Eat! family. ***You've got to see them all!*** *Each video features tasty carbohydrate-rich, dairy-free recipes and a different cookbook. The entire Let's Eat! family is listed below. Ask for them at you local book store. New books and videos are released regularly.*

- ❑ **The Great Sugar Scandal**
- ❑ **Fat...Or Fiction?**
- ❑ **High Protein: Giving Your Bones A Break!**
- ❑ **Digestion: A Churning Question**
- ❑ **Social Drinking: Pleasure Or Prison?**
- ❑ **Food Fixations: Finding Freedom**
- ❑ **Dieting: Victory From the Jaws of Defeat!***
- ❑ **Let's Eat!...Meat?**
- ❑ **MOOOOOve Over Milk***
- ❑ **Calamity In A Cup***

*Award-winning video

(Order form is on page 134.)

Each 60-minute program is just $19.95, plus 10%, or $4.00 (which ever is greater), for S/H. NC residents add 6% sales tax. Better yet, avoid the extra costs, and ask for the tapes at your favorite book store. ***Let's Eat!*** The name people say, three times a day!

It could save you thousands!

IT COULD SAVE YOUR LIFE!

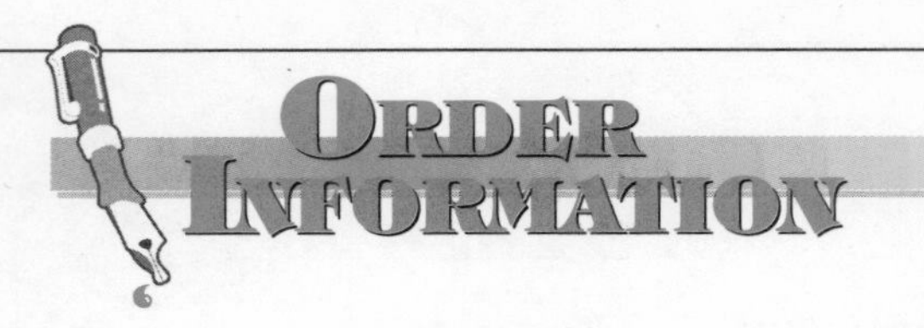

To purchase any of the Let's Eat! cholesterol-free (casein-free!) cooking programs, check at your local book store, or make your selection(s) on page 143, fill in the form below, and mail to:

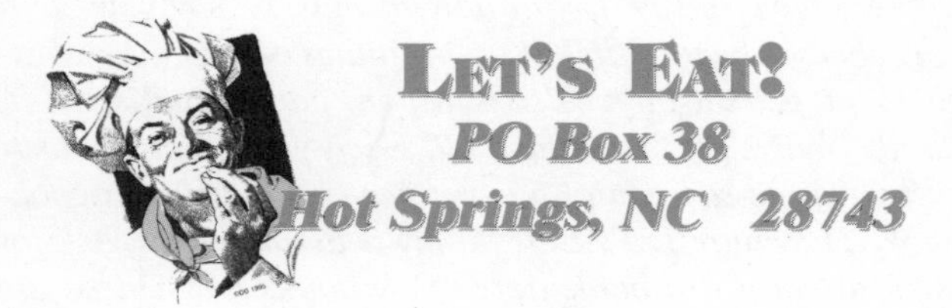

For credit card orders call:

1-800-4-LET'S EAT!

(1-800-453-8732)

Name:____
Address:______________________________________
City:____
State: ____________ **Zip:** ____________________

(Please allow 3-4 weeks for delivery.)

☐ **Please send the FREE recipes from page 125.**

Authors: Vicki B. Griffin, PhD, Dane J. Griffin
Coauthor: Virgil Hulse, MD, MPH
Research coordinator: Phylis Austin
Graphic design/editor/rewrite: Dane J. Griffin
Cover design & art: Larry Moore Design Associates, Orlando, FL